The Mending of Broken Hearts

C.A. Williams

The Empire Publishers publishing
12808 West Airport Blvd Suite 270M Sugar Land, TX 77478

https://empirepublishers.co/about-us

Our books may be purchased in bulk for promotional, educational, or business use.
Please contact The Empire Publishers at +(844) 636-4576, or by email at support@theempirepublishers.com

First Edition 2025

About the Author

C.A. Williams was born in Houston, Texas, during the "go-go" days of the oil boom.

His formative years were difficult. Plagued with allergies and frequent bouts of upper respiratory sickness, Williams was unathletic and extremely myopic and astigmatic, forcing him to wear intractably thick glasses and be the subject of ridicule by his classmates. During that time, he developed resilience and courage, along with the skills that are critical to becoming a good writer- insight, creativity, and the ability to observe and remember life events with compassion, honesty, and sensitivity.

Williams has been exposed to a number of experiences that he later called "less than good." In 1992, his parents divorced after a tumultuous, and occasionally violent, marriage of twenty-eight years. In 2004, he was diagnosed with multiple sclerosis after temporarily going blind in his left eye in a dramatic fashion. In 2016, he became sober after getting fired from a job and battling alcoholism for a number of years. In 2017, Williams' mother was diagnosed with Alzheimer's and Parkinson's Disease, and he helped provide care for her until she passed in 2024.

Professionally, Williams worked as an analyst, portfolio manager, investment advisor, and small business owner for a number of years before becoming a full-time writer and motivational speaker.

Along the way in his journey of life, Williams developed a number of hobbies and interests, which include cycling, hiking, working out, and the occasional golf outing (though he doesn't profess to being good). He also is a fan of classical music, live concerts, and sporting events (Go Cowboys!)

Seeing his way through the experiences he endured, Williams has dedicated his life to inspiring and encouraging others during their darkest hours. He now continues to write heart-felt stories and give speeches around the country and world that let people know, "You CAN and WILL make it through life, and *prosper*."

Williams now lives in the Dallas area with his beloved pets and his partner, Gerry.

This book is dedicated to anyone who has experienced, or is experiencing, generational family trauma. With courage, strength, perseverance, and a lot of hard work you can make it through and not let a difficult past define you.

Acknowledgment

I want to thank Ned Harris, Hera Abbottson, and the entire team at The Empire Publishers. Without them, publishing and promoting this book would have been extremely difficult. Ned and Hera's guidance and encouragement were invaluable, helping me to persevere and trudge on when I felt completely demoralized and like tossing in the towel, giving up, and going back to life as I knew it, which felt less than satisfactory in many ways. Ned and Hera challenged me to own my voice and share my story to inspire others to make it through seemingly impossible circumstances.

I also wish to acknowledge my mother's caregiver, Emma, who came along at a difficult time for the family and me, and became the glue that held a fractured family together.

Press on, keep the faith, and NEVER give up.

Table of Contents

Chapter One

"I've lost confidence in you."

That's how it started.

Tyler Dykisma didn't even blink when he said it. His dark, Middle-Eastern eyes locked on me as if I were a stain on his trophy-polished floor. Dylan sat stiffly to his left, and Emily, the intern, perched on a loveseat like she'd stumbled into the wrong funeral.

At first, I thought maybe I misheard him.

"What?" I asked, my voice catching.

He leaned back, as if enjoying this. "At first, I was impressed with your abilities. Your credentials, that designation you carry… It's so coveted, so respected. But…"

I cut him off. "But what?"

"The mistakes, mainly. I just can't have it. I have a business to run." I didn't want to admit it, but I did feel something pinching in my chest.

That room was a museum of self-congratulation, plaque after plaque, trophies for excellence in sales. Funny how quickly excellence can vanish.

He leaned forward, shaking his head. The rascal was pitying me. "I just couldn't do it anymore." I stared at him, arms crossed, forcing my face to stay blank.

"So, it's time for us to part as friends," he said.

Friends. Right. He reached out his hand as if we were sealing a golf deal, not ending my job. I took it, barely. "Fine," I muttered. "I'll file for unemployment."

That lit him up. His eyebrows shot up. "Why? You have assets. And I'll fight it. I have lawyers."

Of course he did. I glanced at Dylan, who was already wearing the face of someone sitting at a wake. Tyler gestured to him. "Dylan will show you out."

So that was it. Box packed, dignity dented. In the rush, I left behind my calculator, a small, stupid thing, but I wanted it. The strong Christian mother F never sent it back.

"Different playground, different rules," I muttered to myself.

Dylan and I rode the elevator down in silence, a silence that screamed louder than words. Outside, he helped me slide the box into my battered blue Honda Element, the one I bought even though Joanna had wanted me to get the Toyota. Another choice I got wrong. I am pretty good at picking the things nobody would want.

"I wish I'd worked for you instead," I told him, half-smiling.

He sighed. "Me too."

That was the eulogy for my career. I drove home. The ride was long, and longer still in my head. By the time I reached the house, my cats were waiting at the door, innocent, always hungry. And then my phone buzzed. A text.

"Sorry that had to happen. I appreciated all your hard work, Tad. It just wasn't a good fit."

A good fit. Was I a bad pair of shoes? You return to the store, thinking, yeah, not my style. Too rough on the toes. I hope I callused his ego just a little bit if not fully.

I set the phone down, and my eyes drifted to the nightstand. The Smith & Wesson was there, calling me. "Do you want to fire me too?"

I picked it up. Turned it over in my hands. Cold metal against my warm skin. This could all be over in a flash. No more screwups, no more firings, no more not fitting anywhere. One trigger pull, and the whole ugly carousel stops.

I slid the round in. Raised it. The taste of steel touched my tongue, sharp, bitter. I pressed the barrel into my mouth, staring at my reflection.

Maybe this was the right way out. Maybe not.

Death is final, they say. But what if I pulled wrong? What if the bullet exploded sideways, left me alive but mangled, deformed? I couldn't stand that.

You are too good-looking to go down like this… Too vain, even now. But the thought of waking up uglier, broken, still breathing this miserable life? That was worse.

Whatever, I thought. *Enough. Let's end this.*

My finger tightened on the trigger, slowly feeling the shape of my cure of choice. This was it. Soon, forever. I am ending things once and for all. I stood there with the gun in my mouth.

How long had it been? Twenty minutes? Five? Time dissolves in moments like this. Even a Rolex can't tell you how long you've been staring at your own death.

I had a Rolex, by the way. Inherited. Two parts. First the watch, then the band. My old joke, "We were so poor they had to give it in two parts." People used to laugh. Nobody believed it, of course. Because the truth was the opposite.

The Rankins, my mom's side, were the kind of rich people who make you feel like a guest in your own story. Storybook rich. My grandfather grew up on a ten-thousand-acre ranch. His uncle had sixty-six thousand. Sixty-six thousand. That's not a ranch, that's a continent. And yet, somehow, my grandfather's family was considered the "poor branch," forced to go into the movie-theater business to make their own money. Poor Rankins. Lowly ten thousand acres.

I remembered Kitty telling me that. Her voice still had pride in it, even when she said we were the lesser branch.

I was still holding the gun.

My jaw ached from clenching the barrel. I couldn't do it. It was too much, too sudden. My finger hovered over the trigger, but my brain had already fled the room, running into old stories, family trivia, anything but this moment.

I was too scared. Too vain. Too handsome. Pick an excuse. Too consumed by everything bad going on in my life, I had no time for death. This seems like a valid reason not to choose an easy way out. There would be no character development. I am not a reader, just an 'excuser', if that is even a word.

I sighed and stared at the man in the mirror. He stared back, eyes hollow but alive.

After what felt like eternity upon eternity, I slowly lowered the gun. Set it gently in the top drawer of the dresser.

"I will come for you later. Right now, I need some rest; it was a bad day. I have enough time to give you later. I don't ghost my relations." I smiled and closed the drawer.

There is always later, always later.

My mind has a tendency to desert the present the moment things become too real. It's a talent, if you think about it, a pathetic one.

I walked to the couch and grabbed the chipped mug on the side table. The coffee was cold, like everything else in the house. I gulped it down because that's what you do when you want to feel something that isn't the hollow in your chest. It tasted of soaked cardboard and old apologies.

The room hummed; the fridge, the AC, the city not caring, and my head started its usual ritual with noise that wasn't here. Time folded, and I was out. My mind decided that now we were going to discuss my birth; October, late sixties, crystalline Houston sky. C-section because Kitty was small, because everything for her had to be tidy and planned. Two weeks late, a valve that wouldn't close, Dr. Keating saying there'd been complications, the Episcopal Hospital treating you like a piece of porcelain. "Dr. Dennis Coolson looked at you," she told me years later, like that made any difference. As if a famous name could edit the whole script of my life.

Mrs. Stephens, the baby nurse, Emma Lucile, was making sure we had the best two weeks of pampering, gowns, and tiny bottles. Then the name. Tankard. Who names a child Tankard in a city that thinks names are currency? "Call him Tad," they decided, charity toward the boy, but teachers had a day-one ritual of saying the "real" first name loud enough for the classroom to decide. Tankard became a taunt in a heartbeat.

"Tank up!"

"What are you tanking about?" The laughter was an initiation I never wanted. It still rings in my ears.

I remember being small and smart and unathletic and allergic to everything good on a playground schedule. Asthma, allergies, extreme myopia, astigmatism, words doctors wrote down like excuses. While the others ran, I watched from the classroom window, sticky with envy, eating Vanilla Wafers while they had chocolate chip cookies. I came to hate those wafers. They were consolation prizes with a dusting of shame.

They kicked my lunch across the room, spat on my homework, and stomped on my sneakers. Once, I was kicked in the groin so hard I thought the world had split open. Teachers heard it happen and did nothing, those white-knuckled silences at Christian school where virtue was taught but cruelty was allowed to bloom. "Be quiet, Tad. They're gonna hate you," I would tell myself, which is a strange self-preservation method: predict your exile and make peace with it before they can reject you.

Dad, Al, was quick to anger. Tiny infractions turned into something biblical. The Christmas tree incident is a movie in my head: five-year-old me reaching up, the ornament glittering similar to a promise, and the tree bowing under my curiosity. He charged in, and a string of words I still taste echoed off the gray carpet. "You stupid, goddamned son of a…" That one line lodged like glass. It shaped how I spoke to myself for decades: a closed loop that fed on itself.

And now here I was, twenty or five minutes later, I'd lost track again, on a couch that knew my shape too well. The cats jumped up, sniffed at my knee like they wanted to know if I was edible, then settled in as if nothing was strange. On the wall, taped crooked with the cheapness of habit, was a photograph of me at five, all hair and earnestness, standing with boys whose names I haven't used in years. My eyes in the picture seemed younger, as if a mercy lived there once that left when giggles turned to jeers and my mouth learned to shut.

My brain did that thing: when the present demanded action, it shoved me into the archives. It's a trick, an involuntary, self-preserving move. If you can't finish the act, tell a story. If you can't face the scream, replay the first time someone yelled at you and see how small and brittle you felt then. It's rehearsal for staying alive, in a perverse way: distract until the urge dissolves. Distract until the dull, heavy thing on your chest loosens its grip enough for another cup of cold coffee.

When life has been cruel, you tend to grow with this never-ending exhaustion. You feel tired all the time. Mentally tired.

Outside, someone laughed, a woman's voice, bright and careless. For a second, my heart hitch-hiked toward the sound, considering it a lifeline. Maybe that's all it would take: a wrong smile, a stranger who looks through you and chooses to stay. But then the sound swam past, indifferent, and the house swallowed the noise back up.

I sat there, brittle and tired, watching the dust move in the shaft of light. I told myself I'd sleep. I told myself I could always come back to the drawer later and decide for real. "Later" is a comfortable myth. It lets you avoid endings and keeps you in the business of promises you never intend to keep.

Still, the memories weren't exactly tokens of consolation. They felt like an autopsy of how a boy named Tankard turned into a man who thought about how he'd die and then made a to-do list about it. I folded my hands, let the cold mug sit empty on my palm, and pretended to plan the rest of my life as if it wasn't already scripted in the echo of my father's voice.

I stared at the wall, and funny enough, I could feel the gun breathing heavily in its bed. Then, without paying further heed, I was gone, slipped somewhere else. My body was still on the couch, but my mind had already left the room for another episode of mangled nostalgia. It happens. I am used to it now. One minute, I'm here in this house; the next, I'm back in that stifling Houston kitchen, ten years old, watching the clock hit 7:30.

Mom's voice comes first. It always does. "Your father always does this. He was supposed to be home for dinner. No call. Nothing. Didn't even have the decency to call." I can hear the way her voice cracked on *decency*. She was always big on words like that: *decency, respect, class.* The Rankins had those words engraved somewhere in their family crest, I bet.

I can see her now, Kitty, fork clutched in her hand, tapping the edge of her plate. The food's there, peas and carrots burnt at the edges, meat so overdone it could double as a doormat. I remember thinking her cooking always tasted tired, as if she didn't really want to do it. Maybe she didn't. Grandma Rankin cooked like it was a love language; Mom cooked like it was an obligation.

I'm there again, sitting across from her at the table, pushing food around my plate.

"I can't believe Dad didn't call," I say, because that's what I always said.

"Did you know there are children starving in Africa?" she fires back, automatically. It was part of our dinner ritual. And I remember smirking, just a little, and saying, "Well, why don't we just send the food to them?" That line used to feel brave. Now it just sounds childish, something a dumb kid would say to act snarky.

She gets up, turns off the TV.

"But Mama, I was watching that."

"Just leave it off," she says, the way a judge delivers a sentence.

8

And then silence. That suffocating, sticky silence of Houston nights in late summer, thick enough to chew. The kind where even the air conditioner sounds nervous. The clock on the wall is ticking so loud it's almost rude. 7:45.

I remember the way the air felt. Hot and heavy. My skin prickled just thinking about it. Mama sighed and said something about Missouri, about seasons. Four definite ones. As if the weather could save her from loneliness.

"That would be nice," I said, just to fill the space. "I wish we had that here."

My younger brother, Calvin, had already asked to leave the table by then. Smart kid. He got out early, left me to sit in the soup of Mother's sadness. And then she started again, same sermon, different night. "Someday, Tad, when you marry, remember how to treat your wife. Treat her like she's the best thing you've ever had. Treat her with kindness, respect. Don't take some poor, innocent young woman and treat her like this. She doesn't deserve it."

"I promise I won't, Mother," I said it like a vow, like a priest reciting something he didn't believe. She nodded, satisfied for the moment. Then came the inevitable mention of her father, Grandpa Rankin, the saint of her stories. "My father never treated our mom this way. He was so kind, so wonderful. He was a wonderful man."

I can still see her take that long sip of water before she said it. She always did that, pause for effect, as if she were on stage.

"That's good," I told her, meaning it, sort of. Grandpa was kind, sure, but he was also slipping away by then. "I wish I had known him back then."

"You would've loved him," she said. "He was involved in the community, he cared about people. He loved our mother so much. He was a HELLUVA man, you know that? Decent, kind, ambitious." She leaned back, water glass glinting in the kitchen light. I remember thinking how she said *helluva* like it was a hymn.

8:25.

Her voice rising again: "Where is your father? I can't believe he does this!"

Why *did* he do it? Every time. Every single time. I remember sitting there, small fingers tracing the pattern on the tablecloth, wondering if maybe this was just how families worked, waiting, tension, words said too loudly.

8:27.

"When you get older, don't treat some poor, innocent, young girl this way. You have so much to offer, Tad. You're kind, you're smart, you're ambitious. Promise me."

"I promise I won't, Mother." My voice cracked a little, I think. I felt bad for her. Even now, decades later, that pity tastes sour in my mouth. Then, headlights flashed through the window. Tires crunching gravel.

8:29.

That sound in the driveway, the car door, slow and heavy. The steps, not cheerful. No whistle. No paper under the arm.

8:32.

I knew before she did.

"Gonna be one HELLUVA night," I whispered to myself.

10

The memory fades, but not fully. I blink and the walls of my home return, faint and indifferent. The mug's still in my hand. The cats are asleep. But part of me's still at that dinner table, sweat dripping down my back, peas cooling on my plate, waiting for a door to open and chaos to walk in.

Sometimes I think I live more in those rooms than in this one. Maybe that's the real addiction, slipping into the past where everything already hurts, but at least you know when the pain's coming. It's predictable there. Safer even than my reality.

And you know, funny thing about mornings after the storm, they always looked so normal. Dad with his coffee, Mom pretending everything was fine, and me, breaking another pair of glasses just to feel like I existed.

I let out a shaky breath. I could almost hear her voice again, *Promise me, Tad.*

And I did, but promises made in old kitchens don't always survive the years.

Chapter Two

Today looked to be a sick day. But not in the good way, if there ever was a good way.

Jeez. I remember when "sick" just meant you weren't feeling great. Fever, cough, maybe a runny nose. You stayed home, your mom made you soup, and you watched cartoons. Now, "sick" means something's *cool*.

"That's sick, man!"

"Yeah, isn't it great?"

I don't get it. Maybe I don't have enough *riz*, that's the new word for charisma, apparently. Somewhere along the line, the world decided to change meanings without consulting me. Different playground, different rules.

Anyway, this wasn't that kind of sick. This was the *real* kind. The up-all-night kind. The lonely, scrolling-through-dating-sites kind. I don't even know what I was looking for anymore, someone to talk to, someone to fill the silence, someone who wouldn't hang up when things got quiet.

That's when I thought of Dento.

I'd met him during my first stint in AA. Or as I like to call it, my *cameo appearance*. Joined the group for a bit, decided I didn't belong, and graduated early. Everyone clapped, sort of.

Dento was one of those larger-than-life guys. Used to be a Wall Street hotshot, pulling down half a million a year. Then, poof, homeless, Salvation Army, the whole nine yards. If anyone could make rock bottom sound something similar to a motivational seminar, it was him. I guess I was impressed. Who wouldn't be? I mean, I've never made half a mil, not even close, but it takes talent to crash that hard and get back up.

So I'd started calling him on mornings like this, when I hadn't slept and my brain was a blender full of regret and cheap bourbon. I'd call while driving, yeah, yeah, not supposed to, I know, but this was an emergency. Life-threatening, even.

"Man, I don't know what's wrong with me," I told him once. "I stay up all night on these stupid sites. Just trying to find a girlfriend or something."

He'd listen. He was good at that part. The listening. Then he'd say something about *acceptance* or *gratitude* and have to hang up because "something came up." Something was always around the corner for him.

Still, I called him again.

Thing is, I didn't even think I was an alcoholic. Sure, I'd had some… *situations*. Bad police officers who thought my ankles were handcuff training tools. The eighteen-wheeler incident on Central Expressway. The nurse at the hospital saying, "You oughta be glad they didn't get your blood alcohol content." Waking up with alcohol poisoning once or twice. Okay, maybe three times. That near-spinout on the freeway during a first date that turned into a last one. The busted-up carport in L.A. But that's just bad luck, right?

I wasn't an alkie. Just a nice guy with terrible timing. But I figured if AA worked for Dento, maybe there was something there for me. Some secret sauce to fix… whatever this was. So I called him again, and this time, he actually picked up.

"Meet me at the Center," he said.

I did.

13

Because when you're out of options, you'll follow anyone who sounds like they have answers. Even if they're just another lost guy who found a new vocabulary for failure.

Dento was in a good mood. He always was. The kind of cheerfulness that feels as if it's fighting for its life behind the eyes. Not sincere, just well-rehearsed.

"So, tell me what's up, buddy? What happened? I'm so sorry about your job," he said, all empathy and even teeth.

I told him the story, same way you tell a cop you 'didn't see the sign.' A friend came over. You know, one of those friends who you see at parties and who eventually says, "We should hang out sometime," and for reasons that should be studied by science, you say yes.

She came over, we talked, we laughed, and then came the inevitable question, "What do you have to drink?"

Scotch, of course. Always Scotch. And we drank it. It worked out fine, for that week, anyway.

But then the drinking started again, like it always does, in quiet, civilized doses. I'd started counting. That's how I knew I was still in control, because I counted. I let the ice melt, made sure each glass looked like a restraint in liquid form. Nothing says "I'm fine" like rationed self-destruction.

My girlfriend didn't think so.

We were at a party one night when she caught me nursing the same glass for half an hour. "Hey baby, you left your drink on the counter," she said. "Why'd you do that? Don't you want another?"

"No, babe, I'm good."

And then I wasn't.

14

The mistakes started happening again. Only this one cost Tyler Dykisma $3,200, and Tyler didn't think it was charming. "This will be the last time you make such a mistake," he wrote in an email.

He was right. It was the last time. The deal flow stopped, and I could feel it in the silence between phone calls. I could hear the silence whisper, 'you are banished...'

The last Saturday before the firing, when I was still living in the bubble of denial, I decided to "treat myself." Four drinks. Maybe five. The last one was Maker's Mark because if you're going to drown, at least do it with style.

"So, four drinks in a night?" Dento asked, raising his eyebrows. To me, he resembled a priest about to diagnose a sinner.

"Four, maybe five. I don't know. Might've had a beer earlier, but it wasn't a big deal."

He leaned back, the way people do when they're about to sound wise. "Dude, if that's all you had, I think you've got other problems besides alcohol. There's something else going on." And there it was, music to my ears. Someone finally said it. I wasn't an alcoholic. I was something else. Something mysterious, maybe even noble. A tragic figure.

"You're right, Dento," I said. "Thanks, man. Really. You've been great. Sorry, I've been bothering you with all this crap."

Decision made. I wasn't one of them. AA was for the birds.

Two days later, I was sitting in an Al-Anon meeting, where technically, I shouldn't have been. That's what my mind kept whispering, anyway. This wasn't for me. It was for *them*, the ones with the real problem. The alcoholics. The ones who couldn't hold it together.

I was fine. I just had a few other issues. Stress. People problems. Maybe a touch of bad luck. Life had been kicking me around lately, and anyone would drink in my situation. Anyone reasonable, anyway.

That's how my brain worked; it loved a good story that made me look okay. I'd tell myself: *You're not an alcoholic, Tad, you're just coping.* And coping was good, right? Better than breaking.

I kept running these scripts through my head as I walked in, late. Maybe ten minutes past the start. Oh well. Who cared? Silly clocks. Why did everyone make such a big deal about time? If you're late, you're late. In Mexico, you show up half an hour late and they still hand you a drink.

The room was packed, and I had to squeeze into a metal chair in the back. The fluorescent lights buzzed like angry flies, and there was this faint smell of burnt coffee and cheap air freshener. It all felt unreal, like I'd stumbled into La-La Land, or maybe the Twilight Zone.

People were already sharing, and God, the complaining. It never ended.

One woman was talking about her husband's inability to put the bottle down. He'd sober up for a bit, something would happen, and bam, back to drinking. They called it "going back out." Whatever the hell that meant.

Another woman, younger, twitchy, said her husband was on crystal meth. Then someone else talked about her man, who kept "going on the wagon" and falling off again. On and off, on and off, as if he were a damn seesaw. Who the f--k could keep track of that?

And then there was this one woman, I swear I didn't even know how to process it, who said her *wife* was an anorexic

16

alcoholic. I almost laughed. What a combination. Anorexic alcoholic. What a sight that must've been.

What a bunch of winners. Or, more like, whiners. And yet, somewhere in all that noise, one story started to sound vaguely familiar.

This guy, sitting across the room, kind of cute, actually, was talking about his alcoholic husband. The guy had been arrested for public intoxication, which, honestly, was pretty damn hard to do these days in Houston. You practically had to beg for it. But apparently, he couldn't stop. Even while on probation, he managed to find the car keys his husband had hidden, went out drinking, and totaled their brand-new Mercedes.

I remember smirking. *Aww, poor guy.*

Then another woman started talking; her husband was always drinking and raging. Someone else had a binge-drinking wife who'd start and couldn't stop until she landed herself in the ER or jail.

Car wrecks, DUIs, hospitals, firings, blackouts, the stories kept coming. A damn trail of tears that didn't seem to end.

Blackouts.

There it was again. That word.

Why did everyone care so much about blackouts? They weren't a big f--king deal. I'd had hundreds of them, maybe thousands. They happened. You wake up, deal with it, and move on.

What was the big damn deal about blackouts?

Except, halfway through the meeting, something shifted. My shirt started to feel tight around my neck, I kept touching, moving it, and the freaking stories stopped being noise. They took the shape of echoes... Echoes of my own life.

And suddenly my brain, that slick little liar, started throwing me images I didn't ask for.

The last in a series of firings. That night, I wrapped my car around a pole and almost lost my right eye. The deferred adjudicated probation. The DUI I *almost* got the night of my grandmother's funeral. That date that went completely sideways because I was too drunk to remember her name. The wreck in LA when I was too hungover to stand straight. The carport I'd dismantled, literally, because I was still drunk from the night before.

And I sat there thinking, *who the hell am I kidding?*

The meeting ended, and everyone stood, joined hands, forming this big, human chain, and the thoughts came, relentless, pounding.

My exes knew.

My bosses knew.

My probation officer knew.

Hell, even strangers probably knew.

Everyone but me.

And somewhere, beneath the noise, this tiny voice, this last shred of honesty, started screaming:

Tad. Stop lying. You know it. They know it. The whole damn world knows it.

The gig's up.

Put down the f--ing spear.

It's over.

And that was all my delusional brain needed. *Oh my God*, I thought, *I'm the alcoholic they're talking about.*

It landed with a thud so deep it almost hurt. The memories, the regrets, the near-deaths, they all came flooding in. My whole adult life was one giant, messy, chaotic blur.

How the hell had I missed it? How had everyone else seen it but me?

It was all right there. Clear as daylight. Truth was standing in its purest glory, and I felt ashamed to even look at it. It was a horrifying sight, worse than even seeing Al's face after he returned from wherever the hell he was.

My mask fell, and it hurt like a bitch.

When the meeting ended and everyone dropped hands, I stood there for a second too long, like I'd forgotten what to do next. People were chatting quietly, some hugging, others putting on jackets. I grabbed my keys and left without saying a word.

The night outside was colder than I expected. Houston nights always carried that humidity as if the air itself was sweating. My car was parked under a flickering streetlight, and for a split second, I thought about just sitting there. Not starting it. Not doing anything. But I did. I turned the key, and the engine came alive. I pulled out onto the street, and then my mind started spinning.

You idiot. You absolute f--king idiot.

How could you not see it? How could you walk around for years pretending you were fine when every goddamn person around you could smell the truth a mile away?

My hands were gripping the steering wheel so tight that my knuckles turned white. "You're the joke, Tad," I muttered under my breath. "The goddamn punchline."

The dashboard lights glowed that eerie orange, and the road stretched ahead, empty, silent in mock. Streetlights smeared into long, liquid streaks across my windshield.

You had jobs. You had people who trusted you. You had friends who tried to help. And what did you do? You drank them all away, or did you? How do you know what your reality is, you freaking drunk brain?

I could feel it, that familiar burn behind my eyes, not from tears, but from shame. Thick, oily shame that coated everything. The thoughts kept coming at me, missile-shaped. Damn, I hated myself so freaking much. Who needs haters when you've got a brain like mine?

Maybe they were right to fire you. Maybe you were never that smart, never that talented, just lucky enough to fake it for a while. Maybe every good thing you ever had came with an expiration date stamped "Tad's self-destruction."

I laughed and scoffed at the same time. The traffic lights blurred red to green, green to yellow. I wasn't even sure how long I'd been driving.

And then another thought hit, sharp as glass, *what if I don't stop? What if I just keep driving?*

I tightened my grip. Took a slow breath. "No," I whispered. "Not tonight."

I turned down my street. My reflection in the rearview mirror carried a look of a stranger, who was this worn-out guy?

The house came into view, half-dark, porch light still flickering like it had been for weeks. I pulled into the driveway and cut the engine. The silence that followed was deafening. For a long time, I just sat there, both hands still on the wheel, breathing like I'd just run a marathon.

Greater Heights seemed more beautifully loathsome when I was drowning inside my own head.

That small, stubborn voice knocked again. The one that always crawled back up after I'd torn myself down. *You made it home, Tad. You didn't drink. You're still breathing.*

Another had followed it through the hole; it hissed, *'For now.'*

I leaned my head back against the seat, closed my eyes, and tried to quiet both of them. I didn't know whose side I wanted to be on.

When I got home, I called my girlfriend. Voicemail. Of course. Typical. I tossed the phone onto the bed. Maybe some tunes would clear the air. I was feeling melancholy, that heavy kind that sits on your chest like a fat cat you can't push off.

I put on some music, lay back, and stared at the ceiling. My heart wouldn't stop pounding. My body was trying to run a race my brain hadn't signed up for. I barely slept the entire night. Eyes open, heart doing somersaults, brain chewing on itself. I tried to focus on my surroundings, but the house didn't help much; it was a constant poke to the reality of my existence. The bedrooms still smelled faintly of old carpet, even after I'd torn it up with a friend to reveal the wood floors underneath. The dining room window was rotting out from years of moisture, thanks to the neighbor's fence pressed too close against my wall. The paint was chipping, and the bathroom was a sad affair with its cheap plastic tub surround and clogged showerhead. The kitchen's Formica countertops and sagging cabinets had seen better decades, and the hood above the stove wore a permanent film of grease, like old regret. Once upon a time, someone had tried to turn the place into a duplex, two gas connections, a missing door hidden behind a full-length mirror, the ghost of someone else's plan.

When I still had hope, before the Tyler Dykisma incident, I'd spent a little money to fix things up, had the walls painted a soft tan, and laid down fake wood floors over the linoleum. It looked better, in a dim-light, don't-look-too-close kind of way. I moved into the garage apartment to hold onto the house, the rent barely keeping me afloat. Roaches claimed that space like they'd paid the deposit themselves. I'll never forget the sight of that one monster of a cockroach, just crawling up the wall above the kitchen counter like it owned the place. The countertops there were old, tiled relics from the 1940s; cracked, stubborn, and still holding on. Kind of like me.

The next evening, there I was again, back at the goddamn AA meeting. The Center. Didn't wanna be there. Didn't even know why I was there. I walked in late, as usual. Room full of folding chairs, bad coffee, and people pretending they wanted to be there. I scanned the room like I was checking for landmines, then saw someone I knew.

"Hey, Tad! Come over and sit with me."

Roger. Of course, it'd be Roger. I'd known him for years. I forced a smile and sat down beside him. Up front, this guy, Daniel, I think. He was droning on about sponsorship or some shit similar to it.

"Oh, f--k, here we go," I muttered under my breath.

I'd done that whole sponsor thing before. Did I really have to do it again? Couldn't AA just teach people how to *drink better*? I mean, come on, moderation, pacing, hydration, right? Didn't everyone need that? But no, it had to be all or nothing. Abstinence. Sobriety. The fun-killers. And then there were the clichés. Jesus.

"It works if you work it."

"One day at a time."

"If I heard one more f--king cliché…"

I wasn't gonna do anything here but complain, and that's exactly what I did. Roger nudged me and nodded toward Daniel. "He'd be a good sponsor for you."

"Him?" I said. "I don't even know the guy."

But then again, when had that ever stopped me? I'd started hundreds of relationships with people I didn't know, and most ended exactly the way you'd expect. So yeah, why not? One new sponsor, one shiny little desire chip, and boom, the reluctant hero begins his journey.

The steps. Again. Steps I didn't want to take. Didn't think I needed to take. Hadn't I done this stupid dance before?

Yeah. Third time, if we're counting. Each time, I swore I'd never stay, and I didn't. I always managed to find that one passage in the Big Book, the one that says, *"If you can control and enjoy your drinking, you're probably not an alcoholic."*

And I'd cling to that line like a drowning man holding a cocktail umbrella.

See? I'd tell myself. *You can control it. You can enjoy it.*

Except I couldn't. And I knew it. And everyone else knew it, too. People f--king sucked, so bad, but here I was, again. They told me to show up. I had to get that damn paper signed.

"F--k you and good riddance," I muttered under my breath as I scribbled my name on the attendance sheet. "I'll play your little game, clean up, move on, and get back to my great life."

Yeah, sure, Tad. Great plan.

God, I hated being there. I *so* f--king hated it. But the benefits sounded good on paper: job, relationship, stability, all the stuff I didn't have. So, what the hell.

Let's do this, right?

The days dragged by like a bad hangover. I was still reeling from the job loss, financial mess, time mess, and emotional mess, all of it. Lost my job on the 14th. Started 'working the steps' again right after.

Nothing happened. No epiphany. No miracle. Just another painfully slow chapter in the world's longest, dullest book.

Ten days later, my phone rang. I didn't answer. My ringer's always off, my version of self-care. If I can't hear the world calling, maybe it doesn't exist. But something about that day felt different. I don't know why. Maybe it was the silence between rings, maybe it was the way my heart didn't panic when it buzzed.

Perhaps my life was getting better.

Chapter Three

Life can be such a shit show. That's what I was thinking, sitting there on my worn-out sofa in the living room of my small, quaint bungalow tucked away in one of those yet-to-be-discovered pockets of 1920s homes just three miles north of downtown Houston. Quaint, sure. Quiet, sure. Picturesque enough for a realtor's postcard, except for the fact that the guy living inside was slowly coming undone.

Such a freaking shit show.

You go on and on, right? You make it out as best you can, take the punches, do the 'soldier on' thing everyone tells you to do. But sometimes, the punches land before you even see them coming.

I kept replaying that last conversation with Tyler Dykisma in my head. *"I've lost confidence in you."*

"I have lawyers, and I'll fight if you file."

"You have assets. You can sell those."

And now, here I was. Again.

How the hell did this happen, again?

I thought I was through with this kind of shit. I thought I'd finally clawed my way out of the chaos, and yet somehow, I'd managed to circle right back into it.

I dragged myself off the couch and shuffled to the kitchen for coffee. Coffee always worked better than therapy, especially now that I couldn't drink anymore. *Oh well, Tad. It is temporary. All this mayhem will pass, and you'll be back to your life as it was.*

Then I actually laughed.

What life?

I picked up my phone. Voicemail. Huh. That was strange. Maybe a recruiter? But I hadn't sent out any applications. Still, maybe some miracle had happened. Maybe someone had heard about the tragic saga of Tad Jaehrling and wanted to offer me a six-figure job with a 20% bonus and decent benefits.

I pressed play.

"Uh, this message is for Tad Jaehrling. Uhm, my name is Bonnie Simpson, and, uhm, I have your mother. Please give me a call."

My heart just dropped. Not a recruiter. A stranger had my freaking *mother*. What the hell?

I stood there, phone in hand, the words echoing in my skull. *I have your mother.* As if she were a missing package someone found on their porch.

My thoughts spiraled. Who the hell was Bonnie Simpson? What did she want? What had my mom done *now*?

God, Mom. I loved her, of course I did, but I'd grown so tired of being her parent. The woman couldn't change a damn light bulb without making it into an ordeal. The air filters, the alarm batteries, always chirping like some cursed bird from hell. There was always something. Always a call. Always me fixing it. And now this.

I called back. She answered almost immediately.

"Hello, Ms. Simpson? This is Tad Jaehrling. You called about my mother?"

"Oh, yes! Mr. Jaehrling, thank you so much for calling. I have your mother here."

"Uh, thank you? But please, call me Tad. My father's Mr. Jaehrling."

"Oh, of course, Tad. Well, yes, I do have your mother here. What a sweet lady!"

Sweet. Sure. When she wasn't driving me insane. "Okay, thank you," I said slowly, trying to keep my voice steady. She didn't sound like a kidnapper, but still, what was this? "When you say you have my mother there, where exactly is *there?*"

"Well," she said, "it seems your mother got lost and ended up here at my house, in San Felipe."

"San Felipe?"

"Yes, it's a little west of Katy. You've probably never heard of us." She was right. I hadn't.

And I just stood there, gripping the phone, the silence hanging thick. Because somehow this felt like the perfect metaphor for everything lately; me, trying to get my bearings, and the people I loved just wandering off somewhere I couldn't reach.

San Felipe, Texas. A town that time seemed to have forgotten. Two shadows past Houston, thirty miles west of Katy, which was already thirty miles west of the city itself. Pretty much no one I knew had ever heard of it. Hell, until that day, neither had I.

Maybe it had been something once, some forgotten dot that made enough of a blip to get a street named after it in Houston. San Felipe Street. Yeah, I'd driven it plenty of times. Never realized it pointed to a real place. Guess it just never quite happened there. Oh well. Some towns make it. Some don't.

That's life. But what the hell was my mom doing there? Of all places.

I sighed. The road to perdition, it seemed, never ran out of miles.

So, I called my father.

This ought to be fun.

"Hello!" he boomed through the phone, his voice absurdly cheerful, as if he'd just won the lottery or snorted caffeine through a straw. How someone with such a messy, god-awful life could always sound that damn chipper was beyond me. It had to be fake. I knew it was fake.

"Wow, Dad," I said. "You're hurting my ears. You must've had a lot of coffee."

"Come on, Tad, lighten up! I'm just in a good mood! Enjoy yourself! Enjoy! Enjoy!"

Yeah. Sure, Dad. Just like that time you chased me around with a shotgun, threatening to kill me, Mom, and then Calvin in Shreveport. Real mood-lifting memories.

I kept my voice calm. No point picking that fight again. "That's great, Dad," I said. "But we've got a problem. Mom got lost."

"Got lost!"

"Yeah, and I'm serious. Can you please stop whatever you're doing, actually listen, and help me go get her?" There was silence. Long enough to prove I had his attention now.

"What happened?" he finally said. "Tell me, son."

"Well, apparently, Mom got lost on her way to meet some friends for lunch or something. I don't have the whole story, but, bottom line, she got lost."

28

A pause. "That's not good. Where is she?"

I sighed, unraveling the whole thing. Starting with the voicemail from this woman named Bonnie Simpson, who said she had my mom in San Felipe. Dad had actually heard of the place, which was a bit funny. He always had some obscure bit of Texas trivia ready to go.

I took a deep breath and tried to sound rational. "So, will you *please* help me get her? We'll go together in your car, pick her up, and I'll follow you back in hers. We'll get her home safely." He agreed. Small miracles. We met up and headed out to rescue my mom, Katherine Rankin Jaehrling.

Drives with my father were always complicated. On the surface, they were dull: two men in a car talking about politics, oil, and the stock market. But underneath it all was a low hum of something else, disappointment, resentment, history that neither of us wanted to dig up.

We always ended up talking about my mom's side of the family. The Rankins. Their "storied" past. Dad loved reminding me about it, and I, like a fool, used to eat it up.

The Rankins had been *something* back in the day. Texas rich. Old land, old money, old pride. I already mentioned the extravagant past; it's not necessary to rehash it, but yes, when I am with him, we have to go through it again, as if it were an exam, and I might have to write it down.

And you know, years later, when I did the math on that, I nearly cried inside. Holy freakin' shit. That's who we were supposed to be?

The Rankins were a legend down south. They knew politicians, hosted parties for movers and shakers, hell, they *were* the movers and shakers. They had this massive six-thousand-square-foot house by the water, the kind that ends up on the historic registry. They traveled the world. There were even *books* written about them. My uncle Emmett had been friends with the President.

So, what the hell happened to all that?

I still don't know. I've read what I could, pieced together scraps from stories, but all I really know is, it didn't end well. Somewhere along the way, the wheels came off. And there I was, decades later, driving through Texas to pick up my lost mom, wondering how the descendants of that family ended up here, in chaos.

Growing up, our house was a mess of tension and noise, and for a long time, I thought that's just how families were. I didn't know any better. I'd watch other kids, other homes, and realize, slowly, that not everyone lived like this. But as a kid, how would I have known what "normal" even looked like?

We watched *The Love Boat* and *Fantasy Island* every Saturday night. The perfect lives, the smiles, the easy endings, it was so far from my reality that it almost felt cruel. And yet, Mom and Dad both swore their childhoods had been perfect. Idyllic, even. Norman Rockwell-level wholesome. So what the hell happened between their perfect pasts and *this*? How do two people walk out of paradise, find each other, and manage to build such a spectacular mess?

I wasn't buying their stories anymore. Something didn't add up. The Rankins were supposed to be the golden ones, the Texas aristocrats, the dreamers, the doers. But somewhere between their myth and my reality, the dream cracked wide open. And here I was, driving with my eternally cheerful father, chasing down my confused mom, wondering which of us had fallen the farthest.

According to my dad, Al Jaehrling, his old man used to own a garage, aka Jaehrling's Garage. They sold new cars and everything. Apparently, it was a big deal back then, a real family operation in some well-off suburb near Pittsburgh. There were seven kids total. One was stillborn, and they just called him "Baby Jaehrling." The others didn't fare much better. One rolled off the bed when Grandma wasn't looking, and the other caught pneumonia and died. Hard to imagine how easy it was for kids to die back then. I think about that sometimes, the fragility of it all. You blinked, and a life was gone.

Both my parents, Kitty and Al, were the youngest in their families. I used to wonder if that had something to do with how they turned out. Maybe being the baby in the family shaped them somehow. My brother used to say it was tough being the youngest, that you got ignored, forgotten. But I never bought that completely. Being the youngest seemed to have its perks: parents who had more money by then, a little more patience, maybe even a clue or two about how not to screw things up.

Of course, that's probably easy for me to say, I was the oldest. Which, in my case, meant I was the one they practiced on. The prototype. I didn't do anything wrong other than being born first, but it sure felt like I paid for it anyway. My brother, Calvin, got to learn what *not* to do by watching me. Whether it helped him or not, well, that's debatable.

Because I did almost everything wrong. And so did Calvin, to be fair. He just went bigger with it. He was the more rebellious one, especially after Mom and Dad's marriage exploded.

Growing up, I was told their marriage started on a blind date. Sweet story, right? Until you realize it was probably a setup from hell. Literally, somewhere along the line, the Devil must've pulled up a chair and stayed awhile, because that's what it felt like in our house; thick air, heavy energy, the kind that clings to your skin.

Mom once told me, in one of her many "oversharing" moments, that their marriage wasn't consummated on their wedding night. I still remember wanting to crawl out of my own skin when she said that. I don't know what possessed her to tell me that. Maybe it was some twisted version of honesty. Or maybe she just wanted to pass the discomfort along. Either way, it felt like an injustice. That was probably when the Devil joined the family for good. He never really left.

You could *feel* him in that house, always there, getting high over our misery. He was in the silence, in the anger, in the sadness. And I guess he followed me, too. Through school, through every awkward stumble, every cruel joke, every bit of ridicule that came my way at that so-called loving Christian school I went to.

Eventually, someone must've noticed how bad it was, because the teachers suggested my parents get me therapy. Imagine that the same people causing half the trauma, paying for someone else to fix it. But sure enough, they did. I went along with it. Maybe I was hoping someone could make sense of the mess.

Over the years, I saw plenty of therapists. Some tried to help, some made things worse. They'd talk about "cycles" and "patterns," about how pain passed through generations, similar to a damn family heirloom. They weren't wrong. One of them even suggested I try AA, said it might help me with my "clarity" and "self-discipline." What she conveniently *didn't* mention was that going to AA meant never drinking again. Ever.

That part, I found out the hard way.

I still tell that story sometimes, and people laugh, at least, they're supposed to. That's the point. Not everyone gets the humor, but enough do to make it worth telling. The best comics bomb sometimes; that's part of the game. You learn, you steal a few good lines, and you move on.

Anyway, one day I went down to this meeting at the San Felipe Club. Not my first invitation to AA, mind you, but the first I actually took up. They started handing out these little chips, tokens, they called them, for "milestones" in sobriety.

"One month sober!"

Clap, clap, clap.

"Two months sober!"

Clap, clap, clap.

"Three months!"

Clap, clap, clap.

And on and on it went, months, years, decades.

I remember sitting there, confused as hell, wondering what it all meant. I thought maybe it was like drinks, one drink, two drinks, three drinks. That sounded reasonable enough. So after the meeting, I pulled a guy aside who'd just celebrated two years and asked him, dead serious, "So what's this mean exactly? Like… how many drinks are we talking here?"

He looked at me as if I'd just confessed to murder.

"It means we don't drink," he said.

"Ever?"

"Not even one."

That's when I knew AA was not for me.

I let them have their temperance program. That was fine enough for them, but I didn't need it. The therapist didn't like that much when I told her about it. She got that disappointed look, the kind that says, *You're not getting better the way I want you to.* Eventually, she fired me. Took her a while to get there, though. I guess she got tired of me being recalcitrant, as she'd call it. I always thought that was a fancy word for "doesn't take orders well."

Truth is, I'd seen my fair share of therapists over the years. Some meant well, some didn't, some just wanted to feel like heroes. They all saw something wrong in me, *something to fix.* And a few of them actually helped, I'll give them that. But most? They just stared through me, nodding, writing notes, pretending they understood.

One of them, the last one I saw before I got myself fired from my last decent job, told me I'd been "terrorized" by my classmates. *Terrorized.* That's the word she used. True enough, I suppose, but damn if it didn't sting to hear it said out loud. To have someone label your pain like a case file. Like I was Exhibit A in a generational curse. The bedevilment cycle, yeah, that's what it felt like. A damn family plague that wouldn't let up.

And then there were those drives out to the oil wells. My old man, Al, loved those trips. He called himself a "wildcatter." I used to think that sounded cool, some kind of outlaw. But really, it just meant he drilled for oil all over Southeast Texas, poking holes in the pine trees, hoping to strike it rich. He was always chasing "the big one." The deal that was gonna make us. The one that was gonna put us on the map.

I never knew what "it" was supposed to be. Maybe he didn't either. But I figured "it" meant being rich beyond belief, owning a house in River Oaks or Tanglewood, a place with winding driveways and oak-lined streets, the kind of place where the lights at Christmas made you forget your troubles. "It" meant fur coats and silver cutlery, china dishes, expensive jewelry, all the stuff my mom never stopped talking about.

She'd grown up with all that, or so she said. She'd tell me that over and over again, how she used to have all the things we didn't. How she could've still had them if Dad had just "been more of a success." Funny thing is, my father used to say the same damn thing. Said he'd grown up with all that, too. The big house on a hill, until the city bulldozed it for a highway project.

I used to sit there listening to both of them, wondering where the hell all that wealth had gone. If both families had been so damn well off, why didn't it ever trickle down to *us*? Why were we always the ones left scraping by, pretending?

Because that's what we were, pretenders. Always one deal away from "making it." Always chasing a dream that never came. Every time my father said, "This is the one, Tad. This deal's gonna change everything," I'd believe him. And every time, it didn't.

I remember one Thanksgiving, after the Foley's Parade, Dad and I drove through River Oaks. The houses were palaces, lit up like Christmas cards. I pressed my face against the window, watching them glow.

"When are we gonna live here, Dad?" I asked.

"I'm working on it, Tad," he said, sighing. "I'm working on it."

That's what he always said.

We'd go home after that, to our "perfect" Thanksgiving dinner. The silver utensils polished just right, the china laid out, the cloth napkins folded neatly. We put on a show, pretending,

35

we were rich folks ourselves. Turkey, stuffing, mashed potatoes, cranberry sauce, all of it looked the part. The food tasted fine, but the pretending left a sour aftertaste. We were so close. Always so close. But never quite there.

And beneath all that pretending was fear. I'd been afraid of my father for as long as I could remember. The yelling, the name-calling, the sudden outbursts. The gut punch when I was eleven. The chokehold when I was a teenager. There were other things too, things I can't quite remember, but I *feel* them, they are bruises in my memory that never healed right.

Those drives to the oil wells, they weren't just about business. They were sermons. Lessons about manhood, about how the world worked, about how you had to fight to be someone. But I think, deep down, my father wasn't just trying to strike oil. He was trying to strike redemption. Trying to prove to himself that he hadn't failed.

And maybe I was, too.

Because somewhere along the line, I inherited that same sickness, the constant need to be *one deal away*. The belief that if we could just hit it big, everything that hurt would stop hurting. The bullies, the shame, the hollow dinners pretending we were rich, it'd all fade away.

But the deal never came.

And we never stopped pretending.

Calvin always seemed to remember more than I did. Whole scenes, whole nights, his memory was the tape recorder of our childhood, and mine had been half erased. I know the nights were bad. I just can't *see* them anymore. They're like smudges behind glass, I know they're there, but I can't reach through to touch them.

What I do remember is my dad knocking on my door late at night after everything had gone quiet. After the chaos, after the yelling, after Mom's muffled crying. He'd knock softly, like that could undo anything, and ask if he could come in. And what was I supposed to say? No?

So I'd say yes.

He'd come in, sit on the edge of my bed, and then he'd just break. He'd start crying, saying, "I'm so sorry, Tad," over and over, until eventually, he'd lie down next to me. Nothing ever happened besides that, but still, it didn't feel right. It didn't feel normal. There was something *off* about it. And later, Calvin told me he'd had the same experience. Like our father was trying to cry his guilt out through us.

Weirdly enough, the oil wells were my escape. His too, I think. When we went out there, everything changed. It was like we were stepping out of the house and into a movie. The smell of mud and metal, the sound of the drills, the clang of the pipes, it all drowned out the noise from home.

I'd walk the wooden planks that covered the wet, uneven ground, climb the metal stairs, and just watch. Watch the roustabouts drilling. Watch my dad talking to them like he actually belonged. He had a kinship with them, those guys. You could see it. Sometimes, I think he liked them more than he liked me. He wanted me to be one of them, rough, strong, practical. Instead, he got a kid with glasses, no upper body strength, and an obsession with grammar.

Going to the well was like stepping into a different version of him, the one that still believed he could "make it." That there was always one more deal, one more well, one more big strike waiting. There was even something they called a "Christmas tree" in the oil business. Just think about it, a *freaking Christmas tree* in the middle of nowhere, spitting black gold. Only in Texas.

We were driving one day when he turned to me and said, "How do you think she got out here?"

"I don't know, Dad. Who knows? You never know with Mom." I laughed dryly. "I mean, this is crazy. I kind of suspected something when I saw what was going on with Rupert."

He sighed. "Yeah, that's a mess. Let's not talk about it. I haven't been involved in your mom's stuff for over twenty-five years. They told me to stay away, and I did. I never liked Emmett, and he never liked me either. Called me 'oil field trash.'"

"That's awful, Dad," I said automatically as if I hadn't heard that story a dozen times before.

Emmett was long gone by then, ten years dead, give or take. Not that death had improved his reputation. He'd been cruel when he was alive, especially to my father. Maybe that's why Alzheimer's hit him so hard at the end. A kind of poetic justice. Then again, the drinking didn't help either.

I looked out the window. The trees were stripped bare, all brittle and gray, late January, the 25th to be exact. I always remember the exact date of things. Precision's my curse. Always has been.

I've been told that's one of the reasons people find me... well, irritating. I can't help it. I once walked into a convenience store with ten packs of gum, placed a penny on the counter, and said, "I'll take ten, please." The clerk looked at me like I was insane.

"Sir, that'll be a dollar," he said.

I pointed at the label. "It says point ten cents. So that's one-tenth of a cent, right? Ten of them make a penny." He didn't laugh. Nobody ever did.

I wasn't trying to be difficult; I just wanted the math to make sense. Why couldn't people just *get it right?* Grammar, too, "can" versus "may," it's not that hard. I know I go down rabbit holes. Always have. People tell me I miss the point, but maybe the point's just not where they're looking.

My past partners didn't get it either. They said I was too blunt, too much, too picky. Maybe that's why I'm single again. Or maybe they just couldn't handle my version of honesty. I call it candor. They called it "exhausting."

Same difference, I guess.

We turned down a narrow road, then another, and before long, we pulled up to the house and just like that, another chapter of the family circus began.

It was a rambling country home. Big yard. Lots of trees, pecan mostly, now leafless. Peaceful in that way only the country could be, where the air smells faintly of dirt and endings. I couldn't live out there, though. Too far from everything. Too still. I've always needed a certain level of noise, chaos, distraction… anything to keep my brain from circling the drain.

Mom's car, a burgundy Honda Accord, sat under the carport, still as a tomb. The pecan trees stretched behind it, skeletal against the gray sky. Brown leaves littered the driveway. Dad and I knocked on the back door. I remember the muffled sounds, rustling, the scraping of chair legs, then the door opened. A pleasant woman stood there. Gray hair, glasses, kind eyes.

"You must be Tad," she said, smiling, "and Mr. Jaehrling, I assume."

She remembered our names. Points for that.

"Yes, that's us," Dad said, straightening a little. "Al Jaehrling."

"Tad Jaehrling," I added.

"Bonnie," she said, like we were all on equal footing now.

The usual small talk followed, polite smiles, handshakes, those meaningless courtesies that patch the silence between strangers. Then she waved us inside. "Would you like to see your mother? She's right this way."

Mom sat at the breakfast table, a half-drunk cup of coffee in front of her. She looked up and smiled when she saw us. "Oh, Al. Tad. Thank you so much for coming to get me. I don't know what happened."

And then she explained. She'd planned to meet her friends for lunch, the same group she'd been seeing for years. But she'd taken a wrong turn somewhere, couldn't find the street she was looking for, couldn't find her bearings. So, she just kept going. And going. And going. Until she didn't even know what city she was in. Finally, she pulled over near a "nice-looking house in a nice neighborhood" to ask for help.

That's when she called me.

We talked with Ms. Simpson, Bonnie, for a while, exchanged numbers we both knew we'd never use again, and made our polite exit. Dad went in his car; Mom and I took hers.

We went out to eat, of course. That's what we always did. It didn't matter if the occasion was a crisis or a small victory, our answer was always food. Something about sitting in a booth, ordering coffee we didn't need, pretending to be normal for an

40

hour. We'd laugh, say all the "right" things, play the part of a functioning family. Then we'd leave, and the illusion would collapse before we even hit the parking lot.

After dinner, we met up again at Dad's townhouse. The same damn sofa he'd had since forever was still there, followed him from the house during the marriage, through one of his financial implosions, and now into this smaller place.

Dad looked serious. "Kitty," he said, "this is hard, but I'm going to need your car keys." She didn't argue. Just looked at him for a second, sad, knowing, and handed them over. That was it. The end of her independence in a single, quiet motion.

The three of us hugged. There was this heaviness in the room that didn't need words. And as we were leaving, Dad leaned close and whispered, "Call me when you get home. We have a lot to talk about."

I knew what that meant.

The timing couldn't have been worse. First, the firing, Tyler Dykisma, my boss. Such a "kind, benevolent Christian man." (I say that with all the sarcasm it deserves.) Then Mom's situation. And, because bad news travels in threes, Dad's heart gave out. One of his valves had almost completely closed.

"It was down to one millimeter," he told me. "It's supposed to be ten. The doctor said if I don't have surgery right away, I'll be dead within a year."

"Well," I told him, trying to sound calm, "I'm glad they caught it now."

And then that day came.

The folks at AA were sympathetic. They'd all been through their own versions of the same storm. "Taking care of my mother during her last days, those were some of the best days of my life," Dan said once. I didn't know whether to envy or pity him for feeling that way. Others shared similar stories, trying to make sense of loss by romanticizing it.

But me? I was just standing there in the wreckage, ticking boxes in my head.

The Trifecta.

Job loss.

Demented mom.

Father on the edge of dying.

Delicious.

AA got a mouthful when it was my turn to share.

There was hardly a sentence I said back then without a cuss word in it. It was like a verbal tic, a punctuation mark I couldn't live without. In the early days, you'd have to practically decode my shares in AA, parse through the cuss words to find the meaning buried underneath. Weird, considering I'd once been a good church boy. Sunday school, choir, youth group, the whole bit. But that was the eighties, thirty-five damn years ago. I guess I'd developed selective memory loss somewhere along the way. Convenient, really.

I was driving my mom home one day after visiting Dad in the hospital when Janice, my sponsor's sponsor, called. "You know, Tad," she said, in that half-soothing, half-condescending tone she uses, "it's said that everyone has a shitty share when they're just starting out. I think you've just had yours."

I laughed, though part of me wanted to throw the phone out the window. Maybe she was right. Those early days in AA did feel momentous, like I was standing on the edge of something, love, purpose, hell, even a job. Everything was on the brink of happening.

For a minute, I thought about becoming an analyst for a brokerage. Looked like a solid gig, numbers, structure, and a paycheck. But Janice talked me out of it. Said it "wasn't aligned" or something. I listened to her. Still not sure if that was a mistake.

Then I thought about teaching. I liked the idea, helping people learn, feeling like I mattered. But I didn't pass the damn test. That was new for me. I wasn't used to failing. Would've helped if I'd actually studied, but instead, I was too busy "fellowshipping" in AA, drinking coffee, talking about my feelings, pretending I had it all under control.

Eventually, after six months of uncertainty and mounting bills, I landed a job with a big brokerage firm out of the Midwest. I was a financial advisor. Which really meant I was in sales, but still, it was a start. I had an income again.

Getting there wasn't easy. The firing had wrecked me. The timing couldn't have been worse. I remember that day too well, the feeling of freefall as I sat down and stared at the numbers. The mortgage payment: $1,500. Add food, electricity, water, the basics. I looked at my savings: $3,200. Not exactly the six-month emergency fund every financial advisor loves to preach about.

Something was definitely rotten in the state of Texas.

Sure, I had retirement accounts, my own house, and a rent house, both mortgaged, of course. I could've sold one or dipped into the retirement savings. But I'd heard the horror stories. People pulling from their 401(k)s, thinking they were saving themselves, then getting slapped with massive IRS bills. (Or as I liked to call them, the *Internal Revenue Crooks*.)

So, I did neither.

Instead, I filed for unemployment. Tyler Dykisma, my saintly ex-boss, had sworn he'd fight it. "It's a matter of principle," he'd said, in that oh-so-Christian tone of his. And he did fight it. I saw his response, and his wife's, too. Lovely Christian people.

In the end, I won. I got my $1,200 in unemployment. One small victory for the damned. But the bills didn't stop. The mortgage, the utilities, groceries, it all kept coming. My only steady income was rent from the garage apartment behind my house, and that barely covered the electric bill. So I turned to credit cards.

Fifteen thousand dollars later, I was in deeper shit than when I'd started. And then came the IRS, twelve grand for a rent house I'd sold. I'd done what's called a 1031 exchange, thinking I was being clever. But when you sell the property you exchange into, Uncle Sam wants his cut if you don't reinvest. They're good like that.

Eventually, I faced the truth: I couldn't afford my life anymore.

So I rented out my own house and moved into the garage apartment. Two cats in tow. Not exactly a glow-up, but hey, it was shelter. After that, I started spending more time at my mom's place. Kitty needed help, and I needed a soft landing, especially after Dad's heart surgery. (He never stopped talking about that doctor afterward, said he owed the man his life. Probably did.)

For a while, I even stayed in my mom's guest room. Separate twin beds, as if we were in a bad sitcom. I'd lie there at night staring at the ceiling, wondering how the hell it had come to this. Me, middle-aged, unemployed, back home, two cats, sleeping in the same guest room as my father after his surgery.

But that's the thing about rock bottom. You don't really see it coming. You just wake up one day and realize you've been living there for a while. And from the looks of it, my bottom seemed pretty solid; there was no going further.

Fingers crossed.

Chapter Four

I wasn't exactly thrilled about moving back in with my mom. I mean, really, why, after all these years, was I back under the same roof? Mid-forties, no spouse, no kids, no savings worth bragging about. Just me, my cats, and my demented mom.

Sometimes I'd sit there, watching her shuffle through the house, and think, 'Why didn't I have a wife who could've helped me out here?' Someone normal, maybe even stable. But with my track record and temperament, I couldn't exactly blame anyone for not signing up for the long haul. I'd done very little to make myself "husband material."

And Mom, Kitty, she'd always been scatterbrained. Sweet, sure, but trying to get her to find something was asking a fourth grader to solve a physics equation. She'd get flustered, anxious, hands fluttering like she could will the missing object into existence.

Then there was her family. God, that bunch could fight about money like it was a competitive sport. Always clawing for more. Kitty herself wasn't greedy, but she loved the comfort that money provided. And don't even get me started on her sister-in-law, Eleanor Ridly Rankin.

Now, Eleanor was a real piece of work. Depending on who you asked, she was either greedy or a heroine. Personally, I leaned toward greedy. Everyone in Corpus knew Eleanor liked getting her way, and she always did. Rumor had it she had her eyes on Mom's money. As if she needed it. The woman was a millionaire several times over. But there it was, her kids' names, listed in Mom's trust.

Why? Who the hell knew?

Still, when Mom started slipping into dementia, I made it my personal mission to make sure Eleanor didn't get a damn cent. I figured, if anyone was going to get screwed over in this family, it wasn't going to be me. I'd seen enough of that movie already.

I remembered, with absolute disgust, how Eleanor had fought her siblings over their father's estate, something closer to $1.2 million, back in the late eighties or early nineties. A ton of money back then. The whole family went at each other's throats for it. Everyone wanted a bigger slice. It became the soap opera of Corpus Christi.

Naturally, Mom had opinions about it, as did her mother, my uncle, and, of course, me. Calvin stayed out of it, though, smart move if you want to keep your mental health in one piece. He hated confrontation, or maybe he just didn't care. Meanwhile, I, magnanimous benefactor that I am, took it upon myself to fight for my share and, out of brotherly kindness, include Calvin's too. That's what brothers do, right?

So, I got involved. I even dragged Al into it. He was in his eighties then, probably bored, maybe scared, maybe just happy to have a new project. Either way, he didn't resist. I think part of him missed having something to fix. And, of course, I called my lawyer, the same guy who'd helped me dodge a financial bullet years earlier when I sold my business. There'd been this sneaky little clause in the lease that could've kept me on the hook as a guarantor even after I sold the business and terminated the lease. Just think, still being liable for a business you didn't even own anymore. I'd confirmed it with the landlord too, just to be sure, and, sure enough, the previous

47

owner was still listed as a guarantor, which wasn't a good sign. I lost sleep over it. Turned it over and over in my head until I finally called the lawyer again, half-crazed. "What the hell do I do?"

And he, calm as ever, said, "Why don't you just ask the buyer to be the sole guarantor, replacing you and the previous owner?"

Brilliant. Why hadn't I thought of that?

So I did it. The new owner agreed; it was a bargain deal for her anyway, and we had the contract notarized at some local bank. For once in my life, something went smoothly. That same lawyer, I figured, could help me clean up Mom's trust too. Get Eleanor's kids off it. Why not? He was already on my payroll. So, I enlisted him. And we got to work. Meetings in his office, long phone calls, all that legal theater. I threw myself into it as if it were a multimillion-dollar case, when in reality, Mom's trust was worth maybe six hundred thousand bucks total, three hundred of which would've gone to me.

But I didn't see that at the time. I was too wrapped up in the principle of it. Too wrapped up in "winning."

Years later, I'd realize how bad it really got. But at the time, I was just angry and frantic. The checks were coming in, the lawyers were running their mouths, and I was losing my goddamn mind. Every time I called the attorney's office, I wanted answers. And when I didn't get them, I exploded. I didn't think I was being abusive; I thought I was just holding them accountable for their incompetence. Turns out, people don't appreciate being screamed at. Who knew?

Next thing I knew, I got a letter in the mail. It was from the attorney, firing *me* and my mom as clients. The letter said something about "verbal abuse" and "unprofessional conduct." But here's the kicker, it came with a full refund. How often does a lawyer *refund* you? That's when I knew I'd really pissed them off.

It was funny, but the joke didn't last long. Somehow, Mom got hold of the damn check and lost it. Something inside me snapped. "How could you be so stupid?" I asked in disbelief. "What were you thinking? This was important!" I unloaded on her like some rabid beast, spitting venom at the one person who still loved me unconditionally.

She just stood there, small, shaking, apologizing. My mom. The woman who'd raised me, fed me, tolerated my endless bullshit, now cowering before me as a child. I could've broken right then. And I did, inside. I saw myself clearly as a cruel man. The kind who lashes out because it's easier than facing what's really broken.

I knew, deep down, that I'd become my father. Al Jaehrling. The man who could roar a lion's jeer when the threat was far away, but cower behind a door when it was real. I'd seen him do it, that time the drunk construction worker, Rudy, came banging on our door, screaming for a fight. Dad talked big when the TV villains showed up, but when Rudy was right there, flesh and blood, he just tried to calm him down. I remember thinking, *if my father can't even stand up to a bully, how's he going to teach me to?*

And now here I was metamorphosed into his echo.

That night, I was sitting in the red chair in Mom's guest bedroom, my mind spinning with guilt and shame. Then came this soft knock on the door. I didn't want to be bothered. The knock came again. I yanked the door open and barked, "What do you want?"

And there she was. Mom. In her pink bathrobe and slippers, hands raised as if I was about to hit her. God. My heart shattered.

"Oh, Mother, I'm so sorry," I said. "I wasn't going to hit you. I'd never hurt you." I hugged her tight, tighter than I ever had. She trembled in my arms. This woman, who'd given me everything, who was now slipping into dementia, was *afraid of me*.

That image still burns in me. Her eyes, the fear, the apology for something she didn't even do. I realized then that the glaciers inside me, all that frozen rage, were finally melting. And what poured out wasn't anger, it was grief.

What had happened to her? What had happened to *me*?

I didn't have the answers. Still don't. But that night, for the first time in a long time, I saw myself for who I really was, and I wept. And I tried to fix myself, at least with her if not for my own life.

When I was staying with Mom, I started taking her grocery shopping every Saturday afternoon. That became our little ritual, just me and Kitty at HEB. Lord, she *loved* that store. You'd think it was a cathedral the way her eyes lit up when we pulled into the parking lot.

We'd leave her redbrick brownstone, drive down Buffalo Speedway, and pass all those brand-new houses, too big for their lots, too proud for their foundations. I'd make some smartass comment about "new money," she'd roll her eyes, and that's how the ride usually went.

Once inside, we'd fuss at each other the whole damn time. We never used a list; she didn't believe in them, and I kept everything in my head anyway. It mostly worked out, unless I got distracted by stuff *I* wanted. Sometimes I'd look at the cart and think, *maybe we should've bought more healthy stuff for her,* but money was tight, and I was always trying to stretch the dollar.

Still, those HEB trips were good times. We'd wander the aisles, grab the free samples, talk about everything and nothing, politics, family, who pissed us off that week. It felt like old times, before her mind started slipping. If you didn't know she'd gotten lost driving home not long before, you'd think she was perfectly fine.

There was this one day she tried to grab an orange soda from the top shelf, don't ask me why she loved those damn things, and the bottle slipped and hit her right on the head.

"Mother, you should be more careful," I scolded her. "I can get those for you." She just laughed it off. Typical Kitty. Sweet, stubborn, and never convinced she needed help.

And then there was Rupert, that so-called "caregiver" who'd wormed his way into her life after helping her brother, Emmett. Guy had a halo on his head and a hand in everyone's wallet. He insisted she needed "support," which was code for draining her bank account and shipping her off to some godforsaken group home. If it hadn't been for me and Dad stepping in, she'd have lost everything.

Anyway, those grocery runs were our little sanctuary. We'd walk the aisles, feeling everything was fine, smiling at strangers, pretending life was normal. But deep down, we both knew better.

I remember once asking my sponsor, Don, "Hey, is it okay to eat food that's cooked in wine?" I was paranoid about slipping up, even by accident. "Yes, Tad," he said, chuckling. "They cook the alcohol out." I believed him. Mostly.

51

When we'd finally finish shopping, we'd roll the cart through the blazing Houston heat, her old 2013 Burgundy Accord waiting for us in the lot. I'd be on the phone with Don, doing my daily check-in, trying to sound as if I had my shit together while juggling grocery bags. Then came the inevitable battle with that damn car FOB.

"How do you open this thing again?" I'd mutter, pushing random buttons.

"Here," Mom would say, patient as ever, pressing the right button with a smile. "See? It's not that hard."

It took me a while, but I finally learned.

Looking back, I'd give anything to be back in that parking lot with her, the sun beating down, me fumbling with the groceries, her laughing softly beside me. Those Saturdays were ordinary, but they were ours. And I didn't know it then, but they were some of the best moments of my life.

After we were done at HEB, Mom and I would head back down Buffalo Speedway, that stretch of road that somehow held the whole city's story in a few miles. You had the old bungalows from the '20s and '30s, still hanging on with their sagging porches and cracked driveways, right next to those ridiculous "McMansions" that looked like they were built by people allergic to modesty. We'd drive by, me shaking my head, Mom marveling at how everything had changed.

"Can you believe people actually live in those things?" I'd say.

"Well," she'd answer, "someone has to. The world's gone crazy, Tad." And she was right. The world had gone crazy.

Then we'd turn onto her street and into the garage, still talking, sometimes complaining about everything, sometimes about nothing at all. Funny thing is, I didn't realize then how much

I'd miss those little drives. I'd give anything to have just one more of them now.

But nothing ever stays the same. Not a damn thing. You blink and it's gone. One day, you're unpacking groceries with your mom, and the next, you're standing alone in the same kitchen, wondering where all the time went. Things change right in front of your eyes, and you don't even notice until they're already different, and then it's too late.

Once we got into the garage, we'd haul the grocery bags inside, both of us still muttering about how "things should be." I'd start my usual lecture.

"Mother, you really shouldn't be drinking all that orange soda. It's not good for you."

And she'd shoot right back, without missing a beat, "Well, I *like* orange soda, and I'm going to have my orange soda whether you like it or not."

Her pantry was tiny, barely enough space for half the stuff we bought, so putting everything away took some Tetris-level maneuvering. Eventually, we'd get it done. Sometimes, on rare occasions, we'd eat dinner together afterward, just the two of us sitting at her small kitchen table, but most Saturdays, I'd head out again after we finished. I had my commitment at the Center, meeting up with my AA friends for fellowship, and then the meeting after.

I always felt a little guilty leaving her alone. She'd wave me off, say, "Go ahead, Tad. Spend time with your friends. Don't worry about me. I'm just fine here." And I wanted to believe her but as I was driving away, I'd catch myself wondering, *was she really fine?*

It was always a tug-of-war in my head. Stay with Mom, make sure she's okay, or go be with my people at AA, the only place where I didn't feel completely alone. Most of the time, I chose the meeting. Maybe that was selfish. Maybe it was survival.

I still, to this day, don't know if I made the right choice. I tell myself I did and that I needed the fellowship, the connection, the reminder that life didn't end with my failures. But I'll probably never really know the truth until I cross over myself, wherever that is, if there even *is* such a place.

People say we'll all be reunited someday. I like to think that's true, that I'll see her again, orange soda in hand, smiling that patient, knowing smile of hers. But who really knows? Sometimes it feels like we're all just moving on blind faith, hoping, believing, clinging to that tiny spark that keeps us going when the darkness feels a little too close.

Those drives down Buffalo Speedway, those grocery trips, those quiet Saturday nights, they were simple, fleeting, and everything. And I didn't even see it until it was already gone.

Chapter Five

The bass was thumping so hard I could feel it in my chest, crawling up my ribs, into my throat, and then buzzing at the back of my skull. The lights strobed: red, blue, white, and I felt as if my heartbeat was syncing with the sound. This was the time. This was *the* time. The time to let it all out.

I scanned the dance floor, taking in the chaos. Sweat, perfume, the smell of spilled vodka and lime. Bodies moving like they'd been freed from something. I grinned. Thirty-three years old and finally *someone*. A successful investment professional with a big Houston firm, sharp suit, good tan, built body, tall enough to stand out but not tall enough to scare anyone. If only they could see me now, the ones who used to make my life a living hell. The ones who kicked me in the groin in fifth grade and dumped my lunch tray all over the cafeteria floor. The ones who called me "bug eyes" because of those coke-bottle glasses.

Yeah. Look at me now, assholes.

Kick the dust, Tad. Kick the goddamn dust.

I looked over at Raz… Raul, but no one called him that. We'd met at some charity event in River Oaks, a fundraiser for Parkinson's. He was sharp, smart, came from the same kind of twisted childhood as me. We got each other. Since that night, we'd been inseparable, working out, jogging at Memorial Park, weekend camping trips, late-night conversations that started with nothing and ended somewhere between therapy and madness. The crowd was electric. Music was pounding, the air felt alive. Then, out of the corner of my eye, I saw her.

Dark eyes. Tan skin. The kind of woman who knows she's being watched and doesn't mind it one bit. Her gaze locked on mine, and that was all I needed.

"Excuse me for a minute," I murmured into Raz's ear.

He followed my line of sight and smirked. "Good luck, brother."

I winked, straightened my shirt, and stepped off the dance floor. The beat followed me all the way out, *thump, thump, thump*, as if it didn't want to let me go.

******

Monday morning came for my neck pretty soon. "So, how was everyone's weekend?" Jack asked with a half-grin plastered on his face.

Jack Hammerling: tall, slouched, a little too eager to look in control. My boss, technically. Which meant we all had to sit through this ritual. Monday morning meetings, the most useless twenty minutes of my week. I sipped burnt coffee and stared at the table, half-listening as the others recited their perfectly ordinary lives.

Steve went first. "Well, went to the game, then spent some time with Sam and the boys. Got some time for some much-needed rest. Did the yard, then watched football. It was great…"

Kevin, the baby of the group, chimed in next, "Not much, hung out, watched football, and mowed the yard. It was freakin' hot out there. Cindy and I are getting ready for the wedding."

I bit the inside of my cheek. *The wedding. The house. The dog. The backyard barbecues.* Freaking normies. They lived inside the lines, colored neatly, smiled wide for the photos. They didn't even realize they were on autopilot.

Reggie went next. God, Reggie. The man looked sixty but might've been fifty. Cigarette-stained fingers, gray skin, eyes like he'd seen hell and decided to buy property there. "Grabbed Judy and we had dinner and wine with friends, went out on the boat, then worked around the house." He grinned smugly, probably thinking we all wished we had his life.

Jack turned to me. "Tad?"

I was there, but my head was still in the club. The music. The lights. Her eyes. The way my heart had raced when she smiled at me.

"Tad?" Jack's voice came again. "Earth to Tad."

I jerked upright. "Oh… uh, not much. Just laid low. Nothing special. Been reading this book about Warren Buffett. It's really good. Has a lot of insight on this profession..."

Reggie snorted. "Get a life, Tad."

"I *do* have a life, Reggie," I shot back before I could stop myself. "Not everyone needs to go out and get drunk to feel something. We're not all like you."

Reggie glared, and the whole room went still for a second. Jack cleared his throat. "Alright, alright, let's reel it in, guys. We've got a lot to talk about. The market's been crazy. Everyone's watching what the Fed's going to do."

I leaned back in my chair, half-listening again. The words washed over me like static. All I could think about was how fake it all felt, the small talk, the coffee, the laughter. I'd had more life in my veins standing on that dance floor, with the music roaring and the world spinning. Here, it was all fluorescent lights and empty talk.

And I wondered which version of me was real, the one with the drink in his hand and the bass in his blood, or the one sitting here, pretending to care about interest rates.

******

Life was one long, glittering party that never really ended; it just paused sometimes for that monstrous, necessary interruption called *work*. God, even the word made my skin crawl. *Work*. Who came up with that anyway? Whoever it was clearly hadn't discovered vodka tonics and good lighting.

I was a regular on the circuit, the kind of guy people remembered. A rounder, as some would say. I showed up, smiled, shook hands, laughed at the right jokes, and made the rounds. Everyone knew me, and everyone seemed to like me. And yeah, I enjoyed the attention, the smiles, the fake flattery, the way people leaned in just a little closer when they spoke to me. Even when I knew it wasn't sincere. Even when there were strings attached or favors hiding beneath compliments. Didn't matter. I took it all in, fed off it.

After the kind of childhood I had, I *needed* it. I craved it like oxygen. And why not? Things were going great. My career, after a few false starts, had finally found its rhythm. I was no longer the awkward kid with thick glasses and bruised pride; I was a financial analyst at one of Houston's most prestigious investment firms.

The way I got that job was, honestly, the stuff of legend.

Back then, I was stuck in senior management at an adhesive tape company out in The Woodlands. I was good at what I did, but I hated it. There was no thrill in selling tape. I wanted more. I wanted to be *someone*. Francesca, my partner at the time, was *somewhat* supportive, which in her language meant "I don't get it, but whatever, do your thing." It didn't matter either way. Once I set my mind to something, I did it. That was me. Always had been. I didn't wait for permission.

So, I went old school. I picked up *The Book of Lists*, found the top 20 wealth management firms in Houston, and sent each one a letter. A *real* letter. Professional stationery, signature, and all. I told them I'd follow up by phone.

Most didn't care. Some said they'd talk later and never did. But one did.

Someone from a firm downtown agreed to meet.

I walked into that meeting like I owned the place. The Chief Investment Officer, Jack, was sharp, reserved, the kind of guy who measured people in nanoseconds. But that day, I knew I had him. I don't even know what got into me, but I was on. Smooth, confident, a little bit cocky. I could see him weighing me, and I gave him what he wanted to see.

At the end, he asked if I had any questions. I said, "Yeah, how long are you planning to keep looking for someone for this role?"

Jack smiled. "Until I find what I'm looking for."

I held his gaze. "So... have you found what you're looking for?"

He paused. Smiled again. Two days later, the offer came through.

Those were heady days. The kind of days that make you believe in your own myth. I worked hard, studied harder, and played hardest of all. I hit the gym, showed up at every event that mattered, and somehow always found myself in the right circles, the ones that buzzed with money, charm, and the illusion of meaning. I wasn't always the center of attention, but I knew how to hover close enough to the flame to feel its heat. That was something I'd learned the hard way back in my schoolyard years: find the winners, stick with them, and eventually, some of that shine rubs off on you.

But over time, I realized that not every "winner" was worth standing next to. Still, the habit stuck.

When I started studying for my analyst qualification, I promised myself I'd go all in. Three levels, three years. Brutal exams. But I was determined.

Level One, I signed up at the last possible minute in March 2001, staying up until 1 or 2 a.m. most nights just trying to catch up. I passed.

Level Two, the beast. I made a whole study schedule in Excel, color-coded and everything. Studied like a man possessed. Passed that one too.

Then came Level Three. The final boss.

January 2003 rolled around, and I knew what had to be done. Party life went on pause. No more bars. No more late nights. Just me, my books, and the flicker of fluorescent lights at Rice University, my old stomping grounds from MBA days.

I loved studying there. The quiet of those classrooms at night, the way the campus felt like a ghost town after hours, it gave me focus. On weekends, I'd find an empty room and study until the pages blurred.

The exam was the first weekend in June. I'd planned everything. The week before was review time only, practice tests, timed sessions, flashcards, repetition until my brain felt like jelly. I logged every score, every mistake. And, as always, the night before the exam, I took off. That was tradition. Pepperoni pizza from Domino's. No studying. Just rest, a movie maybe, and sleep.

This year was no different. Memorial Day weekend rolled in, and I left the office early. The plan was simple: relax tonight, study all week, crush the exam, celebrate after.

I was driving home, sun dipping low over the city, just thinking about everything, how far I'd come, how much was riding on this. I hit a stoplight and thought of some study material I'd left behind. My pulse jumped. Did I pack it?

Panic hit.

Without thinking, I twisted around in my seat to check the back and felt a little *snap* somewhere in my neck or back or maybe in the universe itself, who knows, and froze. Did something snap? Hmmm. Oh well. I had studying to do.

So, the studying came, and I went to Rice, like I'd always done. The business school, my safe little hole. Maybe I'd see someone there. Maybe not. Hopefully not. It was Saturday morning, and I just wanted peace and caffeine.

I got there, picked a random classroom, set my books down. But first, restroom. My left eye was bothering me. Weird. Was there something *in* my eye? What the hell was happening now? I adjusted my contact and stared in the mirror. That's when I noticed it, a small spot in my left eye. Tiny. Barely anything. But it didn't go away. It grew. And grew. And kept on growing.

It wasn't one of those black spots you see when you're going blind. It was the opposite; it was clear. A bright nothing that just kept expanding.

Later, my buddy Ray came over to cheer me up. He's this aspiring chef, always whipping something up like we're living in a Food Network episode. This time, it was lasagna. Because apparently, carbs fix everything. Didn't he know I was trying to stay hot? But, hell, it was free food, and I liked Ray. Respected him, too.

We sat down, and between bites of lasagna, I told him, "You know, I have this problem with my left eye."

"Oh… what kind of problem?"

"Well," I said, squinting like an idiot, "it's kind of strange. At this point, I have this blank spot in my eye…"

He leaned in, really listening. "It's a blank spot where I can't see. I just can't see. Right now, there's a blank spot where my head's supposed to be."

"Tad, that doesn't sound good. You need to get that checked out."

"I know, Ray, and I promise I will," I said, half-distracted, staring at myself in the mirror again. Why couldn't I see my damn head? It was as if my reflection was evaporating in front of me.

*****

Morning came dark and sticky. The air felt heavy. The world looked strange. Like, half of it wasn't even there anymore. As if someone had erased it with a bad Photoshop tool.

I covered my right eye and peered in the mirror. Holy shit. I couldn't see out of my left eye. At all. I needed to call that doctor. Immediately.

The doctors got me in right away. I've always loved young doctors, so polite, so optimistic, so clueless. They ran through the usual rituals. "Cover your right eye. What do you see? Cover your left eye. What do you see?"

(Why don't we cover *both* eyes and see what *I* see, huh?)

Then came the color tests. "Let's check if you're color-blind." That was it. I lost it.

"How many goddamned times do you need me to tell you I can't see out of my goddamned *left* eye!?"

A collective "oh" swept through the room like a bad sitcom laugh track. A few minutes later, Dr. Hampton came in, clipboard in hand.

"It's your left eye?" he asked. "How long has this been happening? Was it sudden? When did you first notice it?"

Then he came back with the verdict. "Well, I've got news."

"News?"

"You have what's called optic neuritis."

"What? You mean… inflammation of my optic nerve, right?" He nodded.

"Uh, what causes that? Because clearly, it's not very good."

Dr. Hampton explained it: "It's normally caused by one of three things, HIV/AIDS, Lyme disease, or Multiple Sclerosis."

Inside, I was screaming: *I'll take Option B for Lyme Disease, please.*

He went on, "It'll heal itself in time. We'll give you steroids to speed it up."

"That's great," I said, trying to sound upbeat. "Will I get my vision back before the exam? It's this Saturday, you know."

He assured me I would. Perfect. Just in time to bomb the test *with both eyes open.*

My parents showed up later at the clinic. I called them. They were kind enough to take me to lunch.

"I don't want Multiple Sclerosis," I muttered as we walked through the parking lot. "I don't want to be some mumbling, stumbling idiot."

We went to Houston's. The one where the servers have morning inspections, down to their fingernails. It's the kind of place that lets you pretend the world isn't crumbling. Later that day, I went back to the hospital, got my IV steroids, got my vision back, and, believe it or not, took the exam that Saturday.

The morning of the exam, though, my left eye started acting up again. "Oh, shit," I groaned, rushing to the restroom. I leaned into the mirror, heart pounding. And there it was.

"Freaking hell," I whispered. My contact lens was inside out.

*****

So, I began the process of testing.

I didn't have option 1 or 2. Which meant the only one left, the one I'd been pretending didn't exist, had to be 3.

Multiple Sclerosis.

Still, being who I was back then, I waited until the very last month of 2003 to get the damn test. Denial looks good on me, I guess.

All through 2003, I'd gone about my life pretending everything was fine. You know, fake it till you make it, right? Except I was faking it and breaking at the same time. I went on weekend trips with friends, drank like I was trying to pickle myself, and even went hiking at Big Bend in October. Yeah. Hiking. With half a working eye and a brain screaming something's wrong.

There were house parties. Too many. I caroused, laughed too loudly, and acted like nothing was happening inside me. If there were Oscars for pretending you're okay, I would've won mine that year.

Then came December.

That's when I had the spinal tap, the one and only way for doctors to figure out why I'd gone temporarily blind.

The doctor came in holding a needle roughly the size of the one from that crazy doctor in *Cannonball Run*. No exaggeration. I swear I saw the damn thing glint under the fluorescent light like it knew something I didn't. He said he was going to stick it into my spinal column.

I think he numbed me first, but honestly, I don't remember. Trauma has a funny way of erasing details that aren't funny anymore.

I started shaking.

The doctor glanced at me, all calm and clinical, and said, "You're shaking."

To which I responded, "You're sticking a needle in my spinal column."

He didn't laugh. "Okay," he said. "But please, try not to shake."

So I stopped. He finished. I left the office pretending everything was fine again.

That night, I went out with a friend, my best friend at the time. We'd planned it in advance. He tried to talk me out of it.

"Tad," he said, "are you sure you want to go out that night? I mean… that's a pretty serious procedure."

Looking up to him, desperate to seem unfazed, I said, "Sure, we'll definitely go out. We planned it. It'll be fun."

"Okay," he said.

So we did. We went from bar to bar, drifted into a few house parties. And by the end of the night, somehow, we were sitting in the back seat of a car with a dealer, and I was taking Ecstasy.

Yeah. That happened.

I've hesitated to even talk about my drug use because I still want to work, to exist out in the world with some semblance of credibility, but drugs were part of my story. They were part of my coping, or maybe my self-destruction. Depends on how you look at it.

The next day, I woke up with a hangover that felt biblical. It didn't go away. Saturday bled into Sunday, into Monday, into Tuesday. By Tuesday, I couldn't take it anymore. I called the doctor's office and told the nurse, "I still have a headache." (I didn't tell her *why*.)

"You *still* have a headache?" she said, sounding horrified.

"Yes," I said.

"Oh my God," she blurted out. "You're leaking spinal column fluid! You're going to need an emergency blood patch."

So off to the hospital I went, again. They drew blood from my left arm and injected it right back into the point where they'd taken the spinal fluid. A literal patch job. The leaking stopped. And, thankfully, so did the headache.

It was December 23rd, Christmas Eve Eve, as I like to call it. The day before my father's birthday.

*****

A few weeks later, late January, maybe the 28th, I got the call. Or maybe it was the appointment. I remember the date because I was obsessing over my rental property, staring at my calendar like it held all the answers.

The doctor read it flatly: "The test results are consistent with demyelinating disease, commonly called Multiple Sclerosis."

I stared at him. Blank.

"You're showing no emotion," he said.

And I answered truthfully, "I don't know what emotions I'm supposed to show."

And that was it.

That's the moment my life split in two, the *before* and *after*.

That's the day my journey with Multiple Sclerosis officially began.

Three months later, I found out I'd passed the educational requirements to become a financial analyst. Now all that was left was the professional experience.

The life of an investment professional. Half-blind, half-lucky, fully cursed but somehow still moving forward.

Chapter Six

Three weeks later, the first shipment arrived.

Copaxone.

I remember staring at the box like it had just come from another planet. Out of curiosity, I looked up the price without insurance. Over thirty-five hundred dollars. For a box of syringes.

Wasn't this a little overkill? Apparently not.

Eugene, one of my party buddies, the kind of guy who could sniff out fun from two zip codes away, had a take on the situation when I asked him how much I should actually tell the doctors.

"Well, my advice, Tad, is just to tone it down a bit," he said. "Tell the doctor you like to party a little now and then."

I laughed. "Never. I'll never tell the doctors."

Years later, when I requested my medical records, I found out I'd told them *everything*. Every last detail. I must've been feeling generous that day.

Still, the news, this diagnosis, came at me as a freight train would. How was I supposed to deal with something like that? I knew how. Vodka, caffeine, and lots of vitamins. That's how.

It was Rodeo season in Houston, parties everywhere, people pretending life was one long, glamorous photo op, and I was invited to one of them. So, I did what I always did: I showed up. I drank. I laughed. I flirted. I numbed. Then came the drive home.

I remember gripping the steering wheel, eyes burning, heart racing, that old familiar voice in my head whispering, *You're fine. You're untouchable. You're part of the "it" crowd. Nothing can phase you.*

Except everything *was* phasing me. But I didn't let it show. I turned up the music, convinced myself it was just another night, another ride home. I told myself I'd deal with it later. And somehow, I made it home in one piece.

The insanity kept going for a while. There was that one Sunday afternoon when I got too drunk to drive home and ended up taking a bath in a friend's house. Not exactly a proud moment. Somewhere between the steam and the silence, I broke down in tears.

My friend knelt down next to me and said softly, "You needed a release." Maybe I did. I didn't know anymore.

Then came Pride weekend, a big deal in Houston. The city was lit up in happy flames. Everyone who was *anybody* was there. Me included, of course. I wouldn't have missed it. My friends and I threw these lavish parties, glitter, lights, champagne, the works. We told ourselves it was all for a good cause. We were raising money for people with HIV/AIDS. And, in fairness, we were. It *was* a good cause. But it was also an excuse to keep the party rolling, to keep pretending everything was fine.

June 2004 hit hard. That's when I started seeing a therapist who wanted to try something called EMDR. Sounded like some new-age brain-zapping thing, but whatever, I was desperate enough to give it a shot. Somewhere along the way, she started asking questions I didn't want to answer.

"Tad," she said one day, in that slow, deliberate therapist voice, "I've been thinking this for a while. You really don't know who you are. All I can say is, if you don't watch it, you're on your way to becoming a serious alcoholic."

F—k, I thought. *Are you kidding me?* As if there's an "unserious" alcoholic?

She thought I should start an alcohol log, keep track of what I drank every day.

Sure, whatever. I'd humor her. So, I kept this stupid alcohol diary. How ridiculous. As if the act of writing it down made it any less true. And how do you even count the *other* things?

Okay, well, f—k it. No big deal, right?

That's what I told myself. Every single time.

So, it started with that Friday.

A total success. Not that hard. Only seven drinks or was it eight?

And I'd gone to the Museum of Fine Arts, classy, right? and I hadn't gotten stopped, arrested, or killed anybody, so I'd say it worked out pretty well. So, I had NEVER killed anyone from drunk driving, including myself! So, the drink diary was a success.

Day one down. Success.

Well, at least I recorded it. That was the important part.

Tad, you are such a good student! No wonder you've been so successful.

The next day brought a house party, and who knows how many drinks? I didn't f---ing know. Who cared at this point? F---ing drink diary!! Then more, and then oblivion.

71

And there was some commotion when I was trying to extract cash from the ATM during the middle of a blackout. At least, that's what I was told. I didn't remember that much about it, except that it was fun and that's where I wanted to be: nowhere, lost, and free, all at the same time. Only aware of the fact that you're so totally f---ing aware that you had no f---ing idea what was going on. And you loved it that way.

F---ing drink diary can wait 'til Tuesday. I mean, who the f--- is Ms. Schnitzerdoodle, or whatever her f---ing name was, to talk about not drinking? She said she liked a Margarita now and then. So there. So why the f--- couldn't I have one too?

The next day, Sunday, dawned bright and early at 3 PM. Terry woke me up. I'd passed out somewhere else that was not my bed. Again. God, I had to stop doing that.

"Come on, Tad," Terry said. "It's hopping at Urban Beats. They've got good Mimosas, and hot girls."

I cracked one eye open. Damned Terry. "Well, I suppose some of both would be good."

And we were off. And the party never ends, and the road to perdition ends in oblivion. Two Mimosas led to four, then more, then beer, then blackout.

The next day dawned hard. Someone was nudging me. I painfully opened my eyes. Terry again. What the hell was he doing here?

"Wake up, Tad. Didn't you say you had to be at work by 8?"

"Oh, shit. What time is it?"

"About 7:05, but if you shower and get with it, you can still make it."

Oh, shit. Shit, shit, shit, shit, shit, shit...

Oh, Sprite, my stomach hurt. I needed to vomit, but I couldn't. Maybe I did? I didn't know. And a shower. Christ, I smelled.

"GET OUT." I wrote those two words, exactly like that, in my day planner. They summed it up.

It was time to get out of this racket, once and for all. I was going to kill myself.

My mom had told me the same thing once, and she kind of knew the game. She'd taught me the night-before hangover cure, after all. A resolution, coupled with a commitment. The AA Club down the street beckoned. I committed to going, and I did.

"I don't know if I'm an alcoholic or I'm just crazy," I said. "But here I am. I need help."

"It's simple," Jimmy said. "You're both. Welcome aboard." And just like that, Jimmy became my first sponsor.

We worked together for a while. The year went along. It was a magical time in Houston. To begin with, for the first time ever, it snowed on Christmas Day. Galveston, which hadn't seen real snow in decades, saw nearly a foot. Things with the family seemed to be going well. My friends in Houston were supportive of my participation in the program. And that trip to Acapulco to see Ray, who was there on business. Well, that brought pleasure in many ways.

But "aboard" didn't last long.

I couldn't swap out pretty party people for a collection of mid-fifty-somethings who looked like their best days were fossilized in the rearview mirror.

So, in the spring of 2005, I 'graduated.' And things began to get bad, fairly quickly.

See, I had this problem with my mouth. It opened when it shouldn't have, and my employer noticed. I was ornery, recalcitrant, belligerent, and hostile, but passionate, that's what my boss said.

"You're my agitator," Jack told me once. "That's where I see you. I need an agitator, and you're it."

Only, it didn't work. People complained, not to my face, of course. Then there was that time they told me not to attend a planning meeting. "They don't want any investment people," someone said.

Which, of course, meant *me*.

"OK," I said. And went anyway.

And in that meeting, I had a confrontation with Bonita that didn't work out too well. The results were rapid. A week later, I came back from getting coffee and found a note on my desk: *Can I see you for a minute?*

I looked down the hall. Jack's office. Susan was in there. Not a good sign. Then came the hammer.

"I've eliminated your position," Jack said.

My head spun fast. Oh, that means I'll be transferred, right? Placed somewhere else? I'll still have a job?

Susan shredded that illusion. She started talking about my severance package, the "nice thing companies were doing these days."

"The great thing is," she said, "you have $8,000, which will help you out." Jack walked me out. I followed, numb, until I was back at my desk.

"Are you ok?" he asked, handing me a box.

"Yeah, I'm fine." As fine as one can be when they're blasted out the door with a cardboard box holding what's left of their dignity.

Adjustment took some time. Part-time jobs. Unemployment. A little pity, a little panic. A casual acquaintance I'd met through my uncle passed away, heart failure, I think. He was younger than I was. That hit weird.

At the service, I sat there, the hymns blurring into the hum of my own thoughts, and I had an idea.

Why not just stop working for someone? Why keep getting kicked around by people who smile to your face and stab you with a memo? Why not be my own boss? As foolish as it sounded, it kinda made sense.

So, after wrangling and mangling and a whole lot of planning (and drinking), in October 2007, I bought my first business, a tanning salon struggling to survive in a strip mall between a dry cleaner and a donut shop. Not glamorous, but it was mine. I kept on and kept on, day after day.

Along the way, I met someone, Joanne. Sweet girl. Half Korean, half American. Temper like fire, taste to match it. We met in some country bar. She was up there singing a little diddy by Tammy Wynette, all southern charm and heartbreak in denim shorts.

I made the move. "Here's my number. I can get you a full-body massage, done by machine, of course."

Oh, I had the lines. The charisma. The salesman charm. Two days later, she called. Two days after that, she was on my couch, strumming songs on her guitar. The day after that, she moved in, and then came the questions.

"Do you want kids?"

"I want a $15,000 ring from Tiffany's."

"When can we go to Europe?"

"Uh, I don't know," I said. "I just met you. We'll see."

The truth was, I didn't want kids. At all. They stood in the way, and I wasn't about to repeat the mess I grew up in. Funny how that kind of thing loops back around, though, isn't it? Our fights were legendary. Neighbors probably thought we were auditioning for some toxic reality show. The apple doesn't fall far. Eventually, Joanne left. I was on my own again.

Whatever. I was used to it.

If only people could see what a beautiful person I was inside, they'd snatch me up in a heartbeat.

At least, that's what I told myself on the good days. After seven years of sweat, shouting, and a slow crawl to exhaustion, I made the decision: time to sell the business, and sell it, I did.

It was time for a new horizon. A reinvention. Again. It had been a while since I'd been in the game. Eight years and five months, to be exact. But I'd gotten some training, some coaching. I knew how to talk. How to spin my failures into "learning experiences." Didn't even lie about my background this time.

Tyler Dykisma, dark eyes, sharp suit, pulled down his glasses and looked at me like he was reading the fine print of my soul. "So, tell me more about what you've been doing the past eight years," he said.

And I did. Even told him about the arrest, deferred adjudicated probation. Not my proudest, but honesty sells sometimes.

"Not that big of a deal," Tyler said, shrugging. "You just got caught."

That was all I needed to hear. Forgiven. Normalized. Human again. We talked some more, and things seemed good to go. It took me forever to write the thank-you notes. I kept rewriting them, correcting tiny mistakes. Nothing ever felt good enough, like I was rewriting my own worth in ballpoint ink.

A week later, I got the job offer. Not what I was used to, but it was something. $52,000 a year, plus a potential bonus. No health insurance yet, but "coming soon," they said. Seeing nothing else on the horizon, and being too lazy or too scared to look any further, I took it.

All would be good. Right? I went along. Went along. Went along.

Got my licenses. Studied. Worked. Stayed late. Seven o'clock nights, empty office halls, long drives home. That's the thing about working hard: it keeps your demons quiet. Until your demons learn to find their way into that routine. And so it happened.

One night, after another late shift, I got in my car and just sat there. The parking lot lights looked too bright. The silence too loud.

I started driving, I don't even remember where I was headed, I didn't care. Maybe home. Maybe nowhere. The radio was off. My thoughts weren't.

You really think this is going to work? After everything? After the business tanked, after Joanne, after you turned every good thing into a wreck? You're a repeat offender, only this time it's life you're violating.

The road stretched long and empty, and I gripped the steering wheel tighter. I wasn't drunk, not that time, but I was dizzy with myself.

You can't keep this up forever, Tad. You're a ticking clock waiting for the wrong hour.

Streetlights flickered past, washing over me like flashes of memory. The office. The salon. Joanne's laugh before it curdled into yelling. I felt my chest tighten with this deep, low ache that said, *you've been here before.*

I slowed the car, tried to breathe, tried to drown out the noise in my head. Somehow, I made it home like always. That stupid kind of miracle no one applauds you for.

Pulled into the driveway. Turned off the engine. Sat there for a long time, watching the dashboard lights fade. And I thought, maybe tomorrow I'd figure it out, or maybe I'd just keep going because that's what I do. I go along, go along, go along.

Chapter Seven

Now, there was this thing with mom. She liked to be called 'mother' because *"mom"* was, in her words, *"too trashy."* Said it reminded her of the neighbor across the street and that country western song *"And if it don't work out."*

"Mama" was too childish for me. So, we compromised and decided, *Mother.*

She was not happy with her situation. She'd dance angrily around that sumptuous three-story townhouse, ranting as if she were trapped in a gilded cage. "I'm not a cat," she'd say, arms flailing. "I need to get out. I can't believe I'm cooped up here in this house."

And the complaining continued. Day after day. Night after night. I'd been going over there a lot back then, as I was unemployed and all, so time wasn't exactly an obstacle, and the complaining kept rolling like some background music to my stalled life. It kept playing until, one day, it didn't. We were watching the Super Bowl, Kitty and I, laughing about the commercials. For a few minutes, things actually felt light.

Then came the inevitable sigh. "I can't believe I still can't drive," she said. "I'm cooped up here like I'm some kind of prisoner. I feel like I'm in prison. I'm not a cat! Why can't I just go drive and get out?"

I turned to her. "You really want to drive?"

"What?"

"Come on," I said. "You said you want to drive. Let's go."

She blinked, confused. "What are we doing?"

"Just come with me," I said, standing up. "Come, come." I grabbed her hand and pulled her gently along. We walked through the breakfast room, into the garage. I unlocked the car, opened the door, and handed her the keys. Then I slid into the passenger seat.

"You said you wanted to drive," I told her. "So, let's do it. You drive the car, and I'll guide you."

"Tad, what are you doing?"

"You said you wanted to drive, so come on. Open the garage door, and let's go. You can do it. I know you can."

"Tad, I don't think this is a good idea."

"It's a *great* idea," I said, smiling. "And I know you can do it."

Here's the thing: I'd studied this stuff. Dementia. Muscle memory. Short-term memories vanish, but the physical ones, walking, eating, breathing, driving, they stick around for a while, until the end, and this wasn't the end. Well, not yet.

So she did it. Kitty started the car like she'd been doing it every day of her life. She backed out of the garage, steady and sure, and turned onto the street with a flawless sweep. We turned onto Buffalo Speedway.

"You're doing great, Mother," I said.

"Where are we going?" she asked.

"You'll see." I guided her, turn by turn, and we pulled into the parking lot at James Coney Island, her favorizte spot. Chili dogs. Cheese fries. Root beer floats.

Just like old times. Like nothing had changed. Like the road to forever was still open and endless. She smiled at me with her

80

signature smile, which she was famous for, and people used to say I had it too. Funny, the things that stick.

Looking back, I barely remember the food, or the football game, or who won, or the weather, or even the commercials. But I'll never forget that expression on her face. I may have called her "Mother" for years, but in that moment, the walls came down. She was Mom again. We talked about random things. Family, the past, Thanksgiving plans, little things you don't realize you're tucking away as treasures until later.

"Ready to go?" I asked.

"Yes, I'm ready," she said, still smiling.

So we went down the long road of Buffalo Speedway, the sun dipping behind the houses, until we turned onto her street. She opened the gate, eased the car back into the garage like a pro.

And I turned to her. "You did it, Mom. You did it!"

It was the last time Kitty Jaerhling would ever drive. Mama Kitty smiled from ear to ear.

That smile would last a lifetime. And it was worth every second of the risk. Every seemingly crazy, reckless, beautiful minute.

The months that followed passed quickly, at least on the surface. I was in the new job, knocking on people's doors, trying to convince them to become clients. Kitty was fading, her dementia getting worse. Al was pretending to be healthier than he really was, and somehow, we still found ways to laugh.

Kitty had this sterling silver bell, probably a wedding gift or something, that she kept on the table by her chair. After Al's open-heart surgery, he stayed at her house to recover. She promised to "take care of him," which mostly meant ringing that damned bell whenever she wanted something.

"Nurse Kitty!" she'd announce cheerfully, ringing that damn bell as she came into the room. Al, the patient, would grin like she'd just cracked the world's best joke. Those were the light, funny moments. There weren't many. Then came the other kind of moments. The calls.

"Tad, please help me! I'm locked out of the house!"

"What the heck, Mother! How did you do that?"

"I don't know. I just went out to get the paper, and then, the gate shut."

It was pouring rain that day. I was already halfway to losing my mind, but then this loving woman, someone I'd never met before and would never see again, called me.

"I drove by," she said, "and I saw this woman standing outside the gate in the pouring rain. She was crying, 'Help, help!' So, I pulled over and helped. We went to a neighbor's house, and then we called you. She knew your number."

There was something about hearing that from a stranger that hit me. Kitty still remembered *my* number. There were other moments, too.

I stayed with her for a while so I could help out, cut expenses, rent out my own house; I needed the income. It wasn't easy living there, though. Mama would complain constantly about "the people" who came in to reset the microwave or "messed with" the dishwasher.

"They keep moving my things," she'd say, suspicious, like the CIA was hiding in her kitchen drawers.

And every morning, I'd drag myself up at 5:30 to get ready for my 6:30 AM AA meeting. Sometimes I'd barely be out the gate before I'd hear her yelling and see her running out, robe flapping, slippers slapping against the concrete.

She'd pound on the passenger window.

"Did I take my pills?"

If it weren't my mom, it would've been a scene straight out of a horror movie. And I'd feel evil for even thinking that. Eventually, it became painfully clear that Kitty Jaehrling could no longer live alone. So, it was time. Time for the formidable task of finding a place for her.

Al decided he'd take charge of this little operation. He hired a locator, and soon the four of us, Al, Kitty, me, and the locator, were driving all over Houston, touring places that promised "senior living with dignity."

Some provided meals: breakfast, lunch, and dinner. Some didn't. Some had pools and apartment cleaning. Others didn't. Some had an "active, vibrant senior community." Others looked like small, sad motels where hope went to retire. At the end of it all, we landed on a place Kitty had been talking about for ages, one she swore she wanted to go to.

It had everything she said she wanted: trips, a community that sang together, art classes, Bingo nights, the whole nine yards. The place itself had seen better days; a tall glass tower, a community center, a dining hall where they served breakfast, lunch, and dinner every day except Sunday.

There was a common area; marble floors, a waiting space for visitors, and a smaller room off to the side filled with the kind of outdated furniture people from Kitty's generation actually found comforting. A local Methodist church held services there every Sunday.

Once upon a time, it must've been fancy, a real five-star setup. But now, you could see the decline: tarnished brass, dull marble, a whiff of overcooked vegetables hanging in the air. Didn't matter to her. "I love it!" she said, eyes shining, and that was that.

Movers became the theme of the year.

Movers for Kitty, hauling her things from the townhouse to her new apartment. Movers for me, as I shoved my stuff into storage and camped out at her place. Then movers again when I went back to my garage apartment. And again, when I moved back into my house.

"You're always moving, Tad," one of my friends said. "How can you stand it?" I couldn't. But I did.

Movers, movers, movers. It wasn't cheap, either. And, of course, things disappeared. Paintings, mostly. I had two, one from each of a couple of close friends, gone. Just vanished somewhere between Point A and Point B. Then there was a $9,700 painting that had been Kitty's. That one disappeared too, likely sold off cheap by one of those "estate sale" liquidators whose cleaning fees always manage to eat up any profit they supposedly generate.

What a scam. Those were electric times, strange and restless. Then came the election. The big one, 2016. Kitty wanted to vote. She wouldn't stop talking about it. She'd been glued to the news, bless her heart. She didn't know where to go or how to get there, so I decided I'd take her myself. I found a nearby elementary school that was serving as a polling place and got her ready.

It was a *process*.

"Turn right."

"No, your other right."

"Wait, no, that's the wrong building, Mother!" We were spinning in circles, turning and turning, scampering around like two lost squirrels, and both of us could be a bit argumentative. Family trait. But eventually, we found the spot. I helped her up to the check-in table, where they had that big voter authorization pledge. And there she was, Mama Kitty, in her pink sweater, signing her name as if it was the most important thing she'd ever done.

Once again, we'd reached that point, that dangerous little illusion of perpetuity where you convince yourself that maybe, things will never change. But deep down, you always know they do. Even when you're not thinking about it, not paying attention, the world's shifting right under your damn feet.

After we moved Kitty into the facility, visiting her became a ritual. Me, Al, and sometimes, Calvin with his wife and the kids. We'd show up around lunchtime, sit in the dining hall like good family members, trying to pretend everything was normal.

Lunch was always the same setup: salad, main course, dessert, and coffee. Always the coffee. Afterward, we'd head downstairs to the parlor, join in for the Methodist service, and sing. Then we'd go back up to her fifth-floor apartment and put on a Hallmark movie.

She *loved* those movies. God knows why.

To me, they were hokey beyond belief. Pure drivel. The same recycled nonsense every single time, some ruthless businessman or morally questionable guy would blow into town to make a quick buck, only to bump into some poor, beautiful woman with a tragic backstory (usually caused by said ruthless bastard, though she didn't know it yet). Then there'd be that inevitable moment, the eye lock, the background of

85

autumn leaves or softly falling snow, and bam, love at first sight.

Cue the montage of misunderstanding, redemption, and repentance. The guy gives up the deal, gets the girl, cue the music, roll credits. It felt as if every single one of them had watched *The Music Man* and thought, "Yep, let's just copy that."

Still, no matter how much I criticize, it doesn't matter. She loved them. So I sat through them, every time, pretending to care about whatever factory or Christmas cookie plotline was playing that day. I think for her, I let my brain rot, willingly.

And things did stick together for a blink, in one whole piece. And when things are good or even just *okay*, you want them to stay that way. You convince yourself they will. You build routines, memories, patterns, like sandcastles you hope won't wash away. But they always do.

I knew with Mama, things were changing, always for the worse. First, it was the meds. The ones she had weren't cutting it anymore, so they added more. Then came the angry outbursts. Big ones. Enough that the manager had her committed to an asylum for a week. When she came back, she had new pills, "for her temper," they said.

Those pills stayed long after the week was over. Then came the shaking. "Parkinson's," the doctor said, like he was announcing the weather, and with that came even *more* meds. Med upon med upon med.

Al and I did what we could for as long as we could, mostly Al, honestly. But it got to be too much. She needed full-time caregivers. Truth be told, nothing brings families together quite like calamity. Sometimes it ends well. Sometimes it ends badly. Most times, it's a mess of both.

The caregivers... well, that was a saga of its own. They didn't like her much. And she sure as hell didn't like them.

"This one's late."

"This one doesn't care."

"This one's sassy."

"This one's lazy."

She'd grow fond of one, and then she'd disappear. She'd hate another, and that one would stick around forever. It was a revolving door of mismatched personalities and bad attitudes. Until one day, this woman showed up.

"I'm Emma," she said, proudly, hands on her hips. "And I'm here to take care of you."

Her full name was Emmaline Rosa Sanchez. And, for whatever cosmic reason, Emma *clicked* with Kitty. One day, as Emma was getting ready to leave for her next job, Mama looked at her, eyes wide, full of hope, and asked, "Will you be back tomorrow?"

The funny thing is that she'd never asked anyone that before. Emma said she would. And from that day on, it was set. She kept her word. In time, the others faded away, and it was just the two of them, Kitty and Emma.

Meanwhile, I kept trudging along in my own so-called "journey of sobriety."

Sobriety. God, what a word. It wasn't what I'd wanted. Not for a New York minute. Not ever, but there I was, stone sober, watching my mom fade away one memory at a time, and pretending like I was okay with it.

What the hell had I gotten myself into? Couldn't I just have a drink once in a while? It wasn't that bad, after all. Oh yeah, the ISMs, "incredibly short memories," and the YETs, "you're eligible, too." I was so tired of those AA acronyms and their cute, catchy slogans. They made it sound as if we were at some kind of self-improvement camp, not in the trenches of mental breakdown.

But hell, between the hospital visits, a luxury overnight stay at the McLennan County Inn, which came with a complimentary year of monitoring, courtesy of my very own Dallas County Probation Officer, and the car wrecks (plural), I was starting to see their point. There was the one that almost cost me my right eye, a near DUI where my kind ex-sister-in-law talked the cops out of sending me to jail for the night because, get this, we had just buried my grandmother that day. Throw in a completely busted-up career, which could best be described as "well-rounded," and yeah, maybe I was starting to catch on.

Not that I had much of a choice. The "suggestion" had more or less been *forced* on me by this state worker named Marie, one of those overly cheerful, helpful types. She worked in a state program that supposedly helped people diagnosed with disabilities. I was on that list now, thanks to the MS. I just wanted some clarity, something solid to hold onto, but Marie decided I needed "testing."

This was back in the day, before Kitty got lost. Back when she was still driving. Back when our shattered family was still pretending to be fine. We all knew we weren't. Everyone around us knew it, too; they just didn't have the guts to say it out loud.

So, Marie sent me to this downtown psychologist. Supposedly for answers. The building looked like it had been rotting since the 1950s, somewhere in the bad part of town. The guy, Dr.

Quakenbloom, yeah, that was his real name, was an absolute kook. He had one of those oily half-smiles that made you want to keep a hand on your wallet.

He gave me these stupid bubble charts to fill out, like I was back in school taking a multiple-choice test about my sanity.

Questions were lined up in this manner,

"Do you ever feel hopeless?"

"Do you drink to cope?"

"Do you feel others are out to get you?"

Ridiculous. Why the hell was I even doing this? After a few minutes, Dr. Q comes out of his office and says, "I think that's enough."

"But I haven't finished," I tell him.

"That's okay," he replies, with that same calm tone. "I think we've got what we need."

And then, the classic line came, "Why don't you come into my office?"

I already knew where this was going.

"So," he starts, "why don't you tell me about what brought you here?"

I did, at least the version I thought would make me sound reasonably sane. He nodded through it, his pen scratching. Then he paused. "Do you drink?" I swear to God, I almost laughed.

"No," I said. "Not really."

"Why not?"

"Well," I told him, trying to sound casual, "I had some trouble with it when I was younger, so I just decided to stop."

He raised an eyebrow. "What kind of trouble?"

Shit. Really?

"Well, a car wreck or two. I went to jail, and the hospital. Twice."

He jotted that down. "What kind of car wreck?"

"Oh, shit," I muttered. "I ran my car into the back of an 18-wheeler."

"Hmmm," he said, leaning back. "And had you been drinking?"

I wanted to throw the clipboard at him. *Well, no shit, Sherlock. You think I plowed into a semi because I was stone sober and feeling adventurous?* The rest of the conversation was just more of the same. Questions, pauses, judgments hiding behind polite concern. I was dodging bullets left and right, but I could feel I wasn't winning.

Three weeks later, I'm sitting in Marie's office again.

"Let's see what it says," she said cheerfully.

She handed me the list.

1. Major Depressive Disorder

2. Generalized Anxiety Disorder

And then she paused.

"Read number three," she said.

"'Alcoholic in remission,'" I read aloud, grimacing. "So what's that got to do with anything? I don't drink anymore. What's

90

the point of telling me this? Can't we just move on? I need help."

"Uh, no," she said, all calm and bureaucratic. "That's not how it works. If you want us to work with you, you're going to have to work with us. We need you to go to AA."

I stared at her. "Oh crap. Are you serious?"

"Yes, I'm afraid so, Mr. Jaehrling. That's the way it works."

She pulled out a printed spreadsheet. "Pick a meeting and commit to going. You'll need to have it signed and bring it back the next time we sit down together."

I looked at the sheet, reluctant as hell. Rows and rows of meetings, times, and addresses. This was my life now, a goddamn attendance sheet. This really sucked. Left with no choice, I found one. At the Center. I'd been there before.

"Okay, I'll go to this one," I said. It was an 8 p.m. Tuesday meeting in central Houston. Fine. I could do that. So, I committed, every other Tuesday, arriving promptly at 8:30. Yeah, you heard that right.

When I got there, though, I knew right away I didn't fit in. These people were nuts. Probation. Trouble with the law. Some of them homeless. Busted careers. Failed relationships, walking cautionary tales in bad jeans, if you ask me.

One of the guys, Jerry, came over to talk afterward. He had that "I've seen things" look, like he'd been to hell and rented a timeshare. "If you seriously have this problem," he said, "you'll be glad you came."

We chatted for a bit. Nice enough guy. But I was convinced I didn't have "this problem," and I sure as hell wasn't glad I came. Two months later, I drank.

The doorbell rang. Roberta.

We'd been trading pics and texts for a while, going on four years, give or take. Always dancing around whatever this was. Love, lust, boredom, I didn't know.

I opened the door.

"Hey, babe," she said, and gave me a quick smack on the lips. Then, the words that sealed my fate, "Whaddaya have to drink?"

Oh, shit.

"Well, I do have this bourbon. It goes well with Coke."

"Okay, sounds good. Let's do it," she said, smiling that easy smile that made me commit the 'shouldn't haves'.

A few days later, I was sitting on my couch, staring at my phone. Some stupid game. Something about improving your mental acuity, your "response time." I found it ridiculous. You were supposed to race around, fill a coffee cup with creamer, start another, then serve it before time ran out. What the hell was this trying to prove?

I got bored and checked Facebook. Something weird was going on in Italy. They'd shut down the entire country. Wait, what? Italy, shut down? Because of some virus?

They were calling it a coronavirus.

I couldn't help myself. I had to post about it. "I can't believe they'd shut down a whole country because of some stupid virus."

Sally texted me almost immediately. "Tad, it IS serious," she said. "People are dying. That's why they shut down the country. It's going to come here."

Whatever. Fat chance. I scrolled again. New notification. A friend's 30th birthday invite. They were going skydiving. Now *that* sounded fun. Never officially on my bucket list, but I'd thought about it plenty. A few friends said they were going, too. Why not? Couldn't hurt anything.

And the day came.

I met up with my friend at the AA Center, forgot that I said that, and we drove down to the drop zone near Clear Lake. Big open field, clear blue sky, all that good stuff. They handed me reams of paperwork, all the disclaimers, all the "we're not responsible if you die" forms. Basically, it boiled down to: *You might not survive this, sign here.*

It explained this was a "risky activity meant for mostly athletic, fit people." Which, well... I wasn't. Not anymore. Not like I used to be. I looked around. Where the hell were my other friends who said they'd come? Figures.

Then it was time to go up in the plane.

Fourteen thousand feet.

The engine roared, drowning out every second thought I had. The guide was giving his speech, all about safety, risk, what to do if something went wrong. "There's still time to back out," he said.

I looked out the window. The ground was getting smaller, little toy cars darting across the highway, rooftops shrinking beneath a bright Texas sky. It was one of those perfectly crisp February days in Southeast Texas, the kind that almost made you forget what summer felt like. Cool, clean air. A little bite, but nothing serious. Just enough to trick yourself into thinking you had seasons.

The guide glanced at me again. "Okay, last call. Still time to back out if you want."

Even if I was terrified, which I was, I'd never back down. Not in front of these people. I wasn't going to be *that guy*, the one who chickened out at 14,000 feet. The one they'd talk about later in the parking lot. No way.

"Okay," the guide said, and then he shoved me.

Jesus Christ.

It was the craziest goddamn thing I'd ever done. The guide, this overenthusiastic adrenaline junkie strapped to my back, kept trying to yell something in my ear. I wasn't listening. I couldn't. All I could see was the ground, coming at me faster and faster, as if the whole planet had decided to meet me halfway.

"And pull," he shouted, then yanked a rope, and, *whoosh*, the chute opened.

"Having fun?" he hollered over the wind.

Fun? No. Not even close. "Fun" wasn't the word I'd use for plummeting toward my death at terminal velocity.

Then came the glide.

We were floating now, suspended in midair like a pair of idiots who paid good money to cheat death. One of the workers, some woman who clearly did this every day, was floating nearby with a GoPro, snapping pictures. What was this? Disneyland.

"Isn't this fun?" she yelled, all smiles.

Were they trying to torture me?

"Fun!" another one called. "Isn't it?!"

94

No, it wasn't.

We passed over fences, fields, horses, rooftops, trees, all of it rushing up at us. Faster and faster. My stomach was somewhere near the stratosphere. And then, the ground ruptured right into me. We landed hard. I fell to the ground.

"Oh my gosh, are you okay? Let's get you to a place. You did great!" some woman said. Terri? Tammy? I didn't catch her name.

Yeah, I'd thought about doing this for years, and now I've done it. A check off the bucket list. But "fun"? Not a freaking chance. Morbid, death-defying, nauseating, terrifying, *that's* how I'd describe it.

They guided me over to this wooden deck under a little roof. Everyone was talking at me, telling me how great I'd done, how much fun it was, how I should do it again. If one more person said "fun," I was going to punch them in the face. Not that I'm the punching type. At least, not physically.

"Let's go out to eat," Mason said, grinning.

Sure. Why not. Steak and potatoes. Something solid, real, on the ground. We found a steakhouse, the kind with iced tea, salad, and a dessert menu that could choke a horse. Everyone was laughing, replaying their "fun" moments.

"Can't wait to do it again!" Mason said, all cheerful.

He turned to me. "Aren't you doing it again, Tad?"

I smiled. "Oh sure," I said.

I'd rather rip out my toenails one by one.

Still, who knew? I'd always been a little bit insane. That's probably how I'd gotten here in the first place. We wrapped up, and everyone went their separate ways. Mason to his place. Chad, the birthday boy, to his. And me, the cautiously cantankerous celebrant, back to mine.

I dropped onto the sofa and flipped through the channels. TV had become this weird love-hate relationship for me. When I had a few extra bucks, I'd subscribe to cable. When I didn't, I'd cancel it. Right now, I had it, but there wasn't a damn thing worth watching. I turned it off and went to bed. My stomach was still doing somersaults. I felt sick and bone-tired.

Next thing I knew, I was being ripped out of sleep by this shrill ringing. It was 4:30 a.m. at the time. It started as this distant noise, a faint ring I thought was in my dream. Then came the knocking. Over and over.

"W-what is it?" I croaked.

I checked the clock. 4:30.

What the hell?

My bedroom was at the front of the house, another one of Joanna's "bright ideas." Oh right. The closet. This room had the bigger closet. Great tradeoff.

I got up, pulled open the blinds, and saw two figures outside.

"Who is it?" I shouted.

"Tad, it's your brother and Greg!" Calvin's son.

"Mom's in the hospital."

Oh, damn. We talked quickly, the kind of conversation that's all static and panic. The polite thing would've been to let them in, but I didn't think of it. I was too disoriented, too pissed about being woken up before dawn.

96

Mom in the hospital. Again. Hadn't this already happened? We'd just gone through this with her, the clinic, the tests, the meds. Now, another crisis. A thousand problems. A thousand curses. I grumbled and muttered the whole way there, my head pounding with exhaustion and resentment. 4:30 a.m. Or was it 4:32? Who cared. It was too early.

You were a problem in my childhood. You were a problem in my adulthood. And you're a problem now. That's all that ran through my mind. By the time I finally made it to the hospital, it was 10:30. I parked far out in the lot, no close spots left, of course, and trudged in. They were all there: Al, Calvin, Courtney, Greg, and Emma.

And then I saw her. My mom.

Kitty.

Staring off into the distance like she was already halfway somewhere else. It hit me… really hit me, what she'd become. A sad, lonely, scared old woman.

My anger deflated.

A voice bellowed in my head, *"Tad, you are truly an asshole. Your mom is sitting here dying in the hospital, and all you care about is yourself."*

I wasn't even sure who said it. God? The devil? Hell, maybe it was both. Didn't matter. The voice was right. I felt it crawl into my chest and settle there like truth on fire. Maybe I really *was* an asshole. Or a loser. Or a failure. Take your pick, I'd been called all of them, and for so long that I'd started believing it.

And once I believed it, I'd get mad. That quiet, internal, skin-boiling kind of mad. The kind that eats you from the inside. I wasn't proud of it, but I understood it. It reminded me of that old *Incredible Hulk* show with Bill Bixby, when he'd warn

97

people, "Please don't make me angry. You wouldn't like me when I'm angry."

God, I used to love that line. The world would push him, and push him, and then when the rage came out, it was all over. I got it. Completely.

I'd wanted to go *Hulk* on a few people myself; the bullies, the judgmental assholes, the ones who kicked me while I was down. But I never did. I always folded in on myself, swallowed it all down until it became poison.

I thought about Lou Ferrigno, too, the guy who *was* the Hulk. I'd read somewhere that he'd been bullied when he was little, picked on for being scrawny, and that he'd had hearing issues that made it hard for him to communicate. People made him feel small, so he built himself big. He turned all that pain into muscle and power. I admired that. He'd turned what broke him into his armor, and look how that worked out.

He got rich, famous, iconic. Maybe there really *can* be happy endings.

I stayed in that hospital room with Mom, and the rest of them: Al, Calvin, Emma. We talked a little, mostly about what might've happened, what the doctors said, and then we just drifted into small talk. That shallow, meaningless kind. It smooths the edges, keeps you from falling apart.

The drive home was silent. Just me and my thoughts, heavy as lead. No music, no calls, just the hum of the tires and the ache in my chest. By the time I got home, I felt emptied out. I spent the rest of that day just… existing. Lying around, staring at the ceiling, flipping channels, doing nothing. I didn't want to see anyone. Didn't want to think. Didn't want to *feel*.

But feelings have a way of finding you, even when you're hiding.

The next day, I went to work like a ghost, body there, soul somewhere else. I smiled where I had to, answered questions, got through the day. And then I went home, sat down, and just broke.

I hadn't cried in over three and a half years. But that night, I did. I cried for my mom, for all the memories we'd shared, and for all the ones we'd never have. I cried for the family, for all the love we tried to have but never quite managed. I cried because I knew this was it. This was the beginning of the end.

And when the sobs slowed down and my throat burned, I thought, *Is this what they call a spiritual awakening?*

Because it sure as hell didn't feel holy.

Chapter Eight

Kitty was still dining with her neighbors, making small talk, holding court with that sharp tongue and no-filter commentary. Then came the *incident*. She'd gotten mad at someone in the dining hall and slammed her tray on the table. Classic Kitty move. The community director wasn't amused and sent her to an asylum for a week. Changed her meds, calmed her down, for a while, anyway. But then came *that* call, the one that changed everything.

Mom had wandered off the property. Gone missing. Looking for *Al*.

And that's the part that broke me. After everything that bastard put her through, choking her, humiliating her, telling her she was "so dumb she didn't even know she was dumb," she still went looking for him. Stockholm Syndrome? Maybe. Or maybe it was just love's final, delusional echo. I don't know. I never understood it.

When the call came in, I was at work, trying to convince myself that this was the 'crowning moment' of my career. Well, it wasn't. An election had just wrapped, and tensions were high. Half the office was celebrating, the other half wanted to burn the place down. Then came the message from Marjorie Goldblum, the director of Mom's retirement center. She was one of the 'unhappy' ones politically, but she'd always seemed unhappy about everything, especially me. She didn't like me from the start, and I never cared enough to find out why. Probably because I reminded her of someone she hated, maybe her dad, maybe herself. Who knows.

I saw her name flash on my phone and ignored it. Then the voicemail came through, "Tad, I need you to call me right away. It's about your mother, Kitty."

My stomach sank. I called her back. Her voice was sharp, clipped, self-important. "Tad, your mother wandered off the property last night. She's going to need 24-hour care." There it was. The inevitable.

My brain went into logistics mode: money, care options, insurance. I already knew the finances were bad, but I didn't realize *how* bad. Rupert, Mom's 'compassionate caregiver,' had pretty much bled her dry. I later learned he'd been charging her $2,500 a month and his partner another $420 to 'blow out the patio.' For what? Airflow? Jesus.

When Calvin told me what was going on, I called a meeting with Rupert and Calvin at a local diner. "What the hell is this?" I asked.

Rupert smiled, that slimy, confident smile. "Your mom needs someone to help her communicate and do things around the house."

"Our mom is perfectly capable of communicating," I said. "She might need help around the house, but $2,500 a month? Are you serious?"

"It's the market rate," Rupert said, like he was reading from a brochure.

"It's actually half what you're charging," Calvin added, deadpan.

Rupert didn't flinch. "Well, your mother and I have a *special relationship*. I really care about your mother." I wanted to throw my coffee in his face. Instead, I sat there, biting the inside of my cheek. There was no winning this. Mom was stubborn as hell, and if she'd decided Rupert was her savior, then that was that.

"We know she's going to do what she wants," I finally said. "But what happens when she runs out of money?"

"She can stay with us," Rupert said, smiling wider, as if he'd just solved world hunger. Later, Calvin and I talked. We both knew we had to confront her. So, I called her one afternoon after work.

"Mother, this $2,500 you're spending on Rupert, it's unsustainable." She'd clearly been halfway through a bottle of Ernest & Julio Gallo because she snapped.

"This is *my* money, and I can do what I want with it! You stay out of it!" And then she hung up. So, I did. What else could I do?

Fast forward six years, and here we were. Rupert long gone, money nearly gone, and Mom, lost and confused, wandering around looking for the man who'd tried to kill her decades ago. I wanted to say, *I told you so*. God, I wanted to. But what was the point? Nobody listened to me then. They all said I was greedy, that I cared more about inheritance than Mom's well-being. Maybe they were right, maybe not. I don't even know anymore, but she was my mom. I didn't want to see her end up broke and helpless. And now, here we were, exactly where I'd said we'd end up.

Her expenses were through the roof, and the assets were evaporating. Al and I kept arguing about how to handle it, each of us trying to prove we were the responsible one. He and I had always fought, two bulls in a pen. Father and eldest son, destined to clash.

Al decided to hold a 'family meeting' at Mom's apartment; him, me, Mom, and Emma, her new caregiver who'd somehow become the adult in the room. The meeting started civil. It didn't stay that way. Al threw his barbs, I threw mine, Mom just sat there, watching us like we were a bad TV show.

Finally, I lost it. "What are we supposed to *do*, huh? How are we supposed to—"

"We're talking about *your mother*," Emma cut in. The room froze. For the first time, someone had said it plain. She was right. And it wouldn't be the last time she put us in our place, either. So, the decision was made. Mom would stay at the senior center, and Emma would take over as her full-time caregiver.

The chaos quieted, at least for a minute. But for me, that moment, that one sentence from Emma, started something deeper. I began questioning my own motives. Was I really worried about Mom, or was I just worried about losing control or the illusion of it? Was I clinging to my financial fears because they were easier to face than emotional ones? Or maybe, deep down, I was just her son, trying to protect the same woman who cooked for us, washed our clothes, took us to school, patched us up when we screwed up. The woman who'd done her best, even when her best fell short.

And as I sat there, staring at her fragile frame in that senior center off I-10, it hit me, 'this is where we all end up. Someday, someone will be sitting in a room deciding *what to do with me.*'

That night, I couldn't sleep. The veil had torn a little, the delusion that I was in control, that I was different, that I'd somehow outrun mortality. I hadn't. And that realization kept me up until morning.

It was the fall of 2020, that strange, suspended season when the world felt like it was coming apart at the seams. COVID was raging, everyone was angry about something political, and the air itself felt heavy with tension. My brother and I were talking almost every day back then, trying to figure out what the hell to do about Mom. She was slipping fast, memory holes, mood swings, confusion, and Dad was burning out.

I decided to drive down to Houston and check out the senior center, the one with the "memory care" unit. Just saying those words out loud felt like a betrayal. But it was around my birthday, and I figured at least I could combine practicality with self-distraction.

Dad came with me to the visit. We both had our masks on, sitting across from each other in that sterile lobby that smelled of disinfectant and distant despair. The staff were kind enough, but something about the place felt wrong. When we left, neither of us said much until we got into the car.

Dad finally broke the silence.

"If we put her there," he said, "she will die."

There wasn't a shred of doubt in his voice. Just truth.

"I know," I said. "I feel the same way."

That night, I couldn't sleep. The thought of Mom alone in that place haunted me. The next afternoon, we sat in the courtyard outside. The sky was gray, and the trees were losing their leaves, nature shedding, like we were supposed to.

Emma handed me the card, which I have already told you about, the one that said, "Your mom wanted you to have this," she said.

It was a birthday card. Mom had apparently told Emma to make sure I got it. I opened it, started to read aloud, and didn't make it far. It said something like, *You will always be my son, and I love you.*

I tried to finish, but the words hit something deep. My throat locked up. I broke down crying right there in the courtyard. I didn't want to. I hated that kind of public unraveling. But Emma just sat beside me and put her hand on my shoulder. "It's okay," she said softly. "Everything's going to be okay." She meant it, and for a second, I almost believed her.

Emma's smart in ways that aren't loud or flashy. She sees things, people, clearly. Over time, I started calling her "Mom 2." It wasn't a joke, not really. It was an acknowledgment. She stepped in where everything else seemed to be falling apart. Still, the situation was impossible. We couldn't keep things as they were, but we couldn't let go, either. I offered my house. Told Dad Mom could live there, more space, more quiet, and close enough for me to help.

Dad hesitated, then shook his head. "Let's keep things the way they are."

I could see the fatigue behind his eyes. The kind of exhaustion that doesn't come from lack of sleep, but from carrying someone you love as they fade from you in slow motion. I also asked Emma if she would move in with Mom, help her full-time. She said she didn't want to do that. I didn't blame her. It was asking too much.

So, I tried a different angle. I called Ben, the financial advisor, Dad's favorite guy. My father *loved* Ben, thought he was some kind of money whisperer. I asked Ben to run a report on everything: Mom's liquid assets, her house, her annual expenses, and send it to Dad. He said he'd do it, and he did.

A few weeks later, Dad called me.

"Tad, call me back ASAP."

That was his message. Always dramatic. I called him back, half-expecting bad news.

He answered with his usual overly cheerful voice, the kind of optimism that always felt a bit forced.

"Hey Tad!!! How's it going?!"

"Hey Dad," I said, suspicious already. "Got your message. What's up?"

"Hey, yeah, so I've got an idea, if you're open to it." He paused for dramatic effect. "So, Tad, just an idea…" Another pause. Then he dropped it. "Can Kitty move into your house?" I froze. He actually said it.

"Oh my gosh, Dad, that's a great idea!" I blurted out, trying not to sound too eager. The truth is, I'd been hoping he'd say that, but I knew he had to believe it was his idea for it to stick. Looking back, though, I think maybe he knew exactly what he was doing. Maybe he needed *me* to believe I'd convinced him, just like I needed *him* to believe it was his call. We were two stubborn men, circling each other with love disguised as strategy. That's how Mom came to live in my house.

And yes, Emma agreed to move in, too.

For all the complications, I have to admit, things worked out the way they were supposed to. I'd wanted to sell that house for a mint and buy something grander. It's Dallas, after all, where everyone measures worth by square footage and zip code. But life had other plans.

Now, when I walk past the living room and see Mom sitting by the window, or hear Emma humming in the kitchen, I realize something simple but profound: Home isn't the place you buy, it's the people you refuse to abandon.

✳✳✳✳✳✳

The sun was blinding that morning, the kind of brightness that feels almost offensive. I remember thinking, *What the hell is the sun doing shining so damn bright today?* It was Easter Sunday, and I was driving down from Dallas to see my mom, who, at this point, lived in a fog that shifted and cleared like bad radio static.

Emma called her "KK." She always said it as if the nickname were a warm blanket. I guess that was her coping mechanism, to smile through the madness, to stay chipper, because the alternative was too heavy to carry. When I walked in, I could already hear her. "KK! It's time to get up! Wake up, KK! It's time for me to take you a bath!" she chirped, her voice far too cheerful for the hour.

My mom's voice followed, faint, confused. "Uh… what? Who are you?"

"I'm Emma, KK! Good morning! It's time to wake up!"

There was a pause. Then Mom's voice again, soft and bewildered, "Oh. Ok."

It was strange hearing her like that. Every time I came, I had to remind myself, this wasn't the same woman who used to iron my shirts before school or yell at me for breaking another pair of those damned Coke-bottle glasses. This woman was softer, slower, trapped in a maze she couldn't escape from.

Emma was getting her ready for my visit. She said it loudly, like an announcement to the world. "We need to get ready for Tad. Tad's driving all the way from Dallas!"

"Oh, my," Mom said. She sounded delighted and lost at the same time.

"Do you remember Tad?"

"Yes, that's my son," she said, proud for a flicker of a second.

"Yes, KK! You're so smart!" And then she forgot again. I could tell, even from outside the room.

Emma said she'd had a good morning. She'd been calm, talking about the sunlight and how bright it was. But as Emma bathed her, she noticed the scratches again, the bruises, the lacerations on her arms. Mom had taken to scratching herself, something between anxiety and compulsion. I could never figure it out. Maybe it was her way of feeling something in a world that had stopped making sense.

"No, KK," Emma said gently. "You can't scratch there."

But Mom didn't understand. "Why not? It itches."

Emma kept her patience. She always did. She washed her hair, bandaged her arms, helped her into her favorite lavender dress, the one she used to wear every Easter when Dad was alive. I stood outside the doorway for a bit, listening to what they were talking about.

Hearing her confusion turn to faint delight and back to confusion again. I hated it. I hated that she didn't know where she was. That she didn't know *me*. That she thought Emma was a friend who just happened to show up every day. And yet, when she saw me, her eyes lit up for a second.

"Oh, hi, Tad," she said. "It's so good to see you."

"Hi, Mom," I said, trying to smile. "You look beautiful."

"Doesn't your mother look pretty?" Emma said.

"Yes, she looks beautiful," I said. "It's where I get my looks."

Emma laughed. "You're awful."

"Well, humility's my thing," I told her. Mom laughed softly, that same old laugh that used to fill our kitchen when I was a kid. "Tad, you look so nice. What are you doing here?"

"I came to see you, Mom," I said. "It's Easter."

"Oh, my," she said again, her voice small, confused, and sweet. "Is it Easter already?" And just like that, the light in her eyes faded. She looked past me, her attention drifting to something only she could see. I watched her fingers twitch; she wanted to scratch again.

Emma reached over and held her hand. "No, KK. You can't scratch there."

Mom looked down, puzzled. "Why not?"

"Because Tad's here. We don't want him to see you like that," Emma said softly.

Mom nodded, uncertain. She smiled anyway, looking somewhere just to the left of me. "I like this house," she said. "It's such a pretty house." It was actually *my* house. But I don't think she knew that.

Later, Emma set her up with a coloring book, something the doctors had recommended. She liked that. She'd press too hard on the crayons, determined to stay within the lines. It made her happy in the way small things make children happy. And that's what she was now, childlike, drifting between flashes of memory and the long, blank stretches of forgetfulness.

I watched her color a little, and for a while, I forgot everything, too. The years, the fights, the distance. I just saw my mom, alive, still here, sunlight on her face. I remember thinking, '*Maybe this is what survival looks like.* Not triumphant, not clean, just stubbornly breathing.'

And when she looked up again, for the briefest second, she knew me. Really *knew* me. "Tad," she said softly, "it's so good to see you."

And I swear, in that moment, I would've driven from Dallas a hundred times over.

Kitty wasn't too active these days, but she wasn't a vegetable either. Emma made damn sure of that.

She kept Mom busy with little things to 'challenge her brain,' as she'd say. After all, it was her job to keep KK stimulated. And she did it with the same cheerfulness that could either make your heart melt or your teeth grind, depending on the day.

Mornings started slow. After Emma woke her, there'd be breakfast, eggs, maybe a tortilla or two. Sometimes, she'd make quesadillas with just enough cheese to melt but not enough to make her fat. Mom was a debutante once, and debutantes didn't do fat, or so she used to say. She'd violated that rule a time or two, but still clung to it like gospel.

Coffee was off the table. Couldn't stomach it anymore. She'd overdone that too, like she overdid everything: love, shopping, drinking, living. Emma gave her decaf now, told her it was the real thing. Mom never knew the difference.

After breakfast came TV time. She loved the old westerns and the Hallmark Channel. *Gunsmoke. The Rifleman. The Andy Griffith*

Show. Clean, tidy worlds where good people stayed good and bad people got what they deserved.

Sometimes she'd react out loud, "Oh, that's awful!" or "Poor little thing!" Usually about some young Shirley Temple–type girl getting mistreated before the happy ending rolled in. Those stories made her feel safe. They were predictable, perfect, everything her own life had stopped being.

Mom used to tell me and Calvin about her 'magical' younger years; the glamorous days, the parties, the movie theaters they owned, how everyone adored her and her father, her "man about town." Perfect cars, perfect house, perfect furniture, perfect teeth. And Calvin would look at her and say, "If it was all so magical, what happened?"

No answer. There never was.

That's the thing about perfection: it's a drug. It hooks you, then turns on you. I guess that's why she loved those hokey TV shows. They fed her the delusion that life once had order. But reality had chewed her up and spit her out, right into my guest bedroom, surrounded by half-empty bottles of ginger ale and coloring books.

She'd lost most of her money thanks to Rupert, who'd shown her "compassionate care" while draining her dry. Funny how that works. Didn't she see it coming? Didn't she remember what happened to her father? To her brother? How could she not?

Anyway, Emma kept her world spinning with coloring books, TV, and errands. Grocery runs were a big deal. In the early days, Mom would still walk beside the cart, touching everything, reaching for snacks and things she didn't need.

"No, Mama," Emma would say. "No, KK." Mom would pout and put it back like a scolded child.

Later, when walking got harder, Emma switched to one of those electric carts. Mom loved it, said it made her feel "independent." Sometimes, when Emma was tired, she'd let Mom sit on her lap as they rode together through Wal-Mart. People stared. Some smiled. It was absurd, but it worked.

After groceries, they'd stop at McDonald's for ice cream. Vanilla cones. Mom loved ice cream, and so did Emma. I think that was their secret truce, a sugar-coated peace treaty between two women holding each other together.

Emma also took her to senior socials, the kind of church gatherings where retirees dance and drink lukewarm punch while a local band plays Elvis covers. And Mom loved them. She became popular, the kind of woman they missed when she didn't show up. "Missed you, KK!" the cards would say. "Come back soon! We love you!" Emma saved them all in a shoebox.

She also sent me pictures. At first, they irritated me. Why the hell was she sending me pictures of Mom dancing with old men? Was it proof she was doing her job? Was I supposed to frame these?

"Look, everyone, my mom's two-stepping in the church gym. Let's alert the media." But over time, the sarcasm wore off. I started asking for them. "Hey, how's Mom? Got any pictures?" It became a ritual. I'd get one every few weeks, Mom smiling, laughing, alive. I didn't know those pictures would end up being the only ones I had left.

Then came the hospital calls.

112

Mom started choking more. Emma said she couldn't hold food down anymore; her esophagus had shrunk too much. She'd eat, swallow, and then vomit it back up.

Emma would panic and call me while I was working at my *very important job for a very important company serving very important people.*

"Hey Tad, I was hoping I could reach you. Your mom can't hold down her food; she's throwing everything up." But I'd miss the call, buried in meetings and metrics that suddenly seemed stupid when I'd listen to her voicemail later.

It kept happening. Emma got more desperate. And I got more defensive.

Then Calvin called, timidly. He said maybe it was time to transfer Mom's medical power of attorney to him. I was stunned. Why? Because I was hard to reach? Because he thought he could do it better? I didn't say that out loud, though I wanted to. I've learned not everyone deserves access to my unfiltered thoughts, though, to be fair, I still think most of them are worth hearing.

So I said, "Sure. You can have the medical. But I'm not giving up the financial power of attorney. Ever." He agreed. And that was that. Except it didn't fix anything.

A week later, Mom got sick again. Paramedics showed up at the house. They said, "We need to speak to the medical power of attorney."

And so my brother stepped in, holding up the documents. "You've got him," he said.

The paperwork didn't change the fact that I was still losing her, piece by piece, memory by memory. Emma kept her moving, fed, dressed, occupied. But I knew better. I could see the fade coming closer; its shadow kept growing darker.

113

Some days I'd get her on the phone and she'd call me "sweetheart." Some days she'd ask who I was. And every time I hung up, I'd sit in silence, wondering how someone so full of life could end up like this, coloring inside the lines of a world that had already erased her.

Chapter Nine

The situation seemed to be working beautifully for everyone except me. So, painfully admitting the impossibility of my situation, I went back to therapy. It was time to unwind the wreckage of my life. It hadn't worked in so many ways, hell, in *almost every* way, and it was time to try and build some semblance of a life, if that was even possible.

A neighbor, Cathy, had told me about this therapist, Gloria Bonham. "She's helped me out in so many ways," Cathy said. "I think you'd really benefit from talking with her."

So I made the call, and that's how Gloria and I began the process. We talked about everything: my childhood, my mom's declining health, my father's abuse, the years of bullying, and all the brilliant ways I'd tried to handle it.

One day during therapy, Gloria decided we should dig deeper. "Didn't you say your parents drank?" she asked.

I grimaced. "Yeah," I said. "You could say that." She waited. I could tell she wanted me to elaborate.

"A lot," I added finally.

"Tell me about that," she said. "How did that impact you?"

I told her about the fights; the screaming, the glass breaking, the doors slamming, the kind of soundtrack that sticks in your bones. And then I told her about *the secret*.

Gloria leaned in. "The secret?"

I sighed. "Yeah. The big one." It was a long day, and I still remember it vividly. I'd just gotten home from soccer practice, hot, sweaty, dying of thirst. I'd only recently gotten my driver's license and felt like a king pulling into the driveway.

I walked into the kitchen, and there it was, my mom's water glass on the counter. Now, normally, I wouldn't drink after anyone. Germs and all that. But this was Mom. No germs between us, right? So I reached for it.

And she said, "No, no, no, Tad, that's not..." Too late. I took a big gulp. I coughed some of it out and then raced to the sink to spit the rest out.

"Mother, how could you!" I yelled, feeling betrayed and disgusted.

She just looked at me, pained. "I told you not to drink it, Tad," she said quietly. "Now you know. I'm so, so sorry."

Gloria frowned. "So, it wasn't water?"

"No," I said flatly. "And I don't know if it ever had been."

That was the day another illusion shattered. The day I realized the house had been slowly crumbling for a long time, and I'd just noticed the cracks. Later, I confirmed what I already knew. Half-empty Smirnoff bottle, sitting smugly in the liquor cabinet above the counter. So that's why dinner was burned so often.

I remember storming off to my room that night, full of rage and shame and confusion. Mom just stood there, shaking her head sadly, saying nothing. The crumbling house sank a little deeper into the ground that night.

Gloria must've thought she was getting somewhere with me, because the next session she seemed almost excited. It was a cheerful Saturday in March, one of those deceptively nice Houston days when the air smells like spring but you can already feel summer crouching in the bushes, waiting to pounce.

"Let's try something different," she said. "I'd like for us to discuss one of your most painful memories, one that ripped you to the core."

"Um, I really don't want to," I told her. That was my default answer for most things in life. But after some coaxing, I gave in. She smiled that therapist smile, the kind that's equal parts kind and condescending. "So, how are you today, Tad?"

"Well, not that good," I said. "Honestly, I feel like a piece of shit. But hey, the good thing is, I get to tell my story to the group tonight."

"That's great, Tad," she said. "I'm so proud of you."

"Yeah, but I'm just not feeling it today," I said. And then I started unloading my list of grievances: work, family, the usual suspects.

She nodded. "I'm so sorry you've had to go through all this."

Warm words, although, I wanted *movement*.

"So," I said, "are we going to do some trauma work or not? I really need to do some trauma work."

"Okay," she said. "Fair enough. There's this technique called Gestalt therapy. Basically, you take a painful event, a conversation, a fight, something that's stuck in your head, and you relive it, work through it, find closure."

"Great," I said. "I've got a few of those."

She smiled again. "So can you think of one?"

I thought for a moment. "Yeah. But it doesn't involve family. I think I've kind of made peace with my parents. I get now that they were just two broken people doing the best they could."

"But there *is* something that's been bugging me for years," I said.

"There was this guy, Rick Lambert. College. California guy. Drove a red BMW. Big nose. He looked like a frat-boy mix between Barry Manilow and that cliché 'Chad' bully from every bad '80s movie. A little effeminate, a little smug, you know the type."

I could feel my pulse quicken just thinking about it. That moment had replayed in my head more times than I could count.

"We were at this huge house party near campus. Drinks, loud music, beautiful girls, cool people everywhere. I was drunk, of course, and having a great time. Then someone shouted, 'We've been busted!'" Apparently, the neighbors didn't like a bunch of loud college kids partying all night. So everyone scattered, rushing to their cars.

I jumped into Rick's red BMW, thinking nothing of it, and that's when he stopped cold. "Wait a minute," he said. "Who just got in the car?" A couple of voices mumbled.

"No," he said again, louder. "Who the hell got in the car?"

I spoke up. "Uh, Tad."

"Tad?"

"Yeah." And then he said it.

"Get the fuck out of the car."

I froze. "What?"

He glared at me, every syllable a slap.

"I said, get out of the fucking car."

"But, Rick, the party's been busted, and the cops are here! How am I gonna get home?"

"I don't give a fuck, Tad. That's your problem. Get out of the fucking car!"

"But, Rick?"

"Look, Tad, you're horrible! Get OUT OF MY FUCKING CAR, NOW!"

Yeah. That's what he said. Word for word. I can still hear it, even now, that tone, that finality, like he was doing me some big goddamn favor by letting me exist in his airspace for as long as he had.

Gloria just stared at me after I said it. I swear I saw tears forming, which was weird because, what the hell, therapists weren't supposed to cry, were they?

"So, Tad," she asked softly, "what did you do?"

What did I do? I did what I was told. Like I always did. I got out of the damn car. Stood there like an idiot while Rick peeled out. Then I sat around the house for a while, feeling like a kicked dog. Eventually, I got a ride back to the bar where everyone hung out on Saturday nights. And that's when I decided, screw this. I was done being everyone's punchline. I went right up to Rick and said, "What's up, man? What the hell was that about? You left me there."

He looked at me through those weaselly little eyes of his. "Look, Tad, you're horrible. Can't you see that? Nobody likes you. Everyone avoids you. I mean, why can't you just do everyone a favor and quit hanging around so much? It's

GLARINGLY OBVIOUS you don't belong." A tear rolled down Gloria's cheek then, no mistaking it this time. So maybe therapists *did* cry. Guess I just hadn't earned that privilege before.

"That must have hurt," she said.

"It was devastating," I told her. "I spent the whole rest of the night mourning, commiserating, trying to figure out what the hell I'd done to deserve that. I even called my uncle later, asked what I might've done to provoke Rick."

My uncle, in his infinite wisdom, said maybe I had done something. "Some people are just assholes," he told me. "Keep your head down and they won't hurt you." Not exactly Hallmark advice. And yeah, that hurt too. So, I kept my head down. I buried it all and made a vow, someday I'd be richer, more successful than Rick Lambert ever dreamed of being. But those words stuck. They crawled under my skin and joined the other voices that had been living there rent-free for years; *you're stupid, you're not good enough, you're a dork, you're a loser.* A whole goddamn choir of rejection singing in harmony.

I'll admit, though, I found a bit of satisfaction later on when Rick mouthed off to the wrong guy at the bar and spent the next semester in a sling. Karma, baby. I didn't console him. Just watched, triumphant. I did end up inviting him to my graduation party, stupidly, but I'd hated that motherfucker ever since that night. Still, I forgave him eventually. Not for him, for me. Even if he spent the next few years kissing my rich uncle's ass every time he wanted something.

I don't even know what happened to Rick after that or to most of those people. I've looked some of them up on Facebook; none of them sent a friend request, and neither did I.

At some point, Gloria had me do this exercise. Said it would 'release the anger.' She told me to imagine Rick sitting in the chair in front of me. So, I grabbed a pillow and started pounding it as if it was his smug little face.

"Go to hell, Rick Lambert!!! Go to hell!!!" I kept shouting until my arms burned. Then I stopped. The room got real quiet. I stood up, wiped my face, and grabbed a Kleenex from the box on her coffee table, hanging it to her on my way out. "Here," I said. "I think you need this more than me. I've let it go."

But of course, I hadn't.

Because in my head, I was still saying it: *Go to hell, you goddamned, worthless, weaselly-eyed motherfucker, Richard Bonham Lambert. Go to hell. May you sleep with the scorpions.*

Rick joined the long parade of shitty people in my life, the ones better off left for dead. Just names in yearbooks I'd tossed years ago. Ghosts from a time I pretend doesn't exist. They once existed. Now, they don't or maybe they still do, tucked somewhere inside, whispering every so often. Because the pain never really goes away. You just bury it, let it rot, and hope something good grows in the space it leaves behind. Sometimes it works. Sometimes it doesn't.

Gloria wasn't done. "Tell me more about the drinking and the drugs, Tad. I need to hear more. What made you behave the way you did? What led to that thing with Rick Lambert?"

Oh, shit. Again? Really?

As if throwing up all over my dorm room, ending up in the hospital for alcohol poisoning, getting hauled to jail, and doing deferred adjudicated probation wasn't enough, she wanted *more.*

And yeah, there was more.

It was a cool day in Dallas. I was living there by then, licking my wounds after Vanderbilt. "2.62!" My dad had barked, eyes wide like I'd just confessed to arson. "I can't believe we're paying for this!" Yeah, well, joke's on you, Dad. You weren't paying a dime. Grandma Rankin was footing the bill. But sure, keep up the delusion if it helps you sleep at night, Al Jaehrling.

So, I transferred to SMU. Social life at Vandy had been a disaster. You try puking all over your dorm and coming back from the hospital to find your entire bedroom relocated to the men's bathroom by some smartass, while you're out with a girl who looks like Phoebe Cates.

You g-ddamned motherfucker. I should've punched you, but you bragged about knowing martial arts and being 'super smart,' so I let it go. But Phoebe... oh, Phoebe... If only, if only. Whole damn cities of denial are built on "if onlys."

Anyway. There was this big fraternity event at the Dallas Country Club that night. The kind of thing where brothers and alumni show up in their best blazers, and everyone pretends to like each other. Important people would be there, and I, ever the outsider, was desperate for an edge. So, I went.

Had a few drinks. Vodka Sevens? Cape Cods? Who knows. Three or four, maybe more. Strong ones. I needed that buzz to feel like I belonged, even for a minute.

After the party, I planned to meet my old friend from Houston at his parents' place in Dallas. He'd just wrapped up his first year at Baylor. Good guy. We were going to hit another party, maybe South Fork Ranch, maybe something for Texas-OU weekend. I can't remember now. All I knew was, it was big. The kind of thing where everyone who ever thought they were better than me would be there.

And I still wanted to impress them. Those same guys who hated me almost as much as I hated them. They hated that I spent time with my Houston friend, too. He was athletic, good-looking, confident, everything I wasn't. But I liked having him around. He made me feel safe. Like maybe if someone tried to fuck with me again, I wouldn't have to fold.

I drank at the Country Club, went back to the frat house, changed, and got in my car.

And as I hit Central Expressway, that whisper in my brain started up…

You shouldn't be driving.

Yeah, no kidding. But I did anyway. Because part of me didn't give a damn. Maybe I had a death wish. I blasted down the freeway, New Order on the stereo, weaving in and out of traffic.
Didn't care. Didn't think. Didn't feel.

Catch me if you can, motherfuckers, I thought. *I wanna freaking die. Maybe if I crash, you'll finally notice me.*

How fucking fast could I go?

By the time I pulled into Tom's parents' neighborhood, my nerves were shot. It was one of those quiet, perfect Dallas suburbs, green lawns, tidy mailboxes, golden porch lights. I remember thinking, *God, why couldn't I have grown up like this?* Tom's family: Bart, Bev, Susie, and their dog, Bruiser, were so normal. So calm. They didn't know what chaos looked like.

I said hi, tried to act sober, and made small talk. Then I went to the bathroom near Tom's room, which was on the far side of the house, away from everyone else. And that's when I heard it.

123

Bev's whisper, "Make sure you're driving."

At the time, I wondered if I was supposed to hear it. Maybe she wanted me to hear it. Maybe that's how people tell the truth, quietly, sideways. I've heard that kind of "whisper" before. Not meant to start a fight, but meant to *land*. Either way, I let Tom drive. It was the right call. It meant I could drink more. And I did.

We hit the party. Beer after beer after beer. Someone once told me, "Liquor before beer, you're in the clear. Beer before liquor, never been sicker." So I figured I was safe.

I couldn't tell you how much I drank that night if you paid me. I think we went to South Fork. Maybe downtown. Maybe both. Faces blurred together, most of them people who couldn't stand me anyway.

By the time we got back to Tom's, it was late. He gave me that look and said, "Why don't you stay here tonight, Tad? It's not safe to drive."

"I'm fine, buddy. Trust me. I'll call you in the morning."

"Please, Tad. *Please.*"

"Tom. I'm fine."

We stared at each other for a beat. I hated losing, especially to him.

"Okay," he said finally. "Just… be safe."

"Yeah," I said. "Sure."

Then I drove off. Through the quiet neighborhood, onto the freeway, back toward the frat house I hated but tolerated because, hell, it was a roof. I remember seeing a McDonald's sign glowing like a beacon up ahead. A Quarter Pounder with cheese sounded perfect. Maybe the grease would soak up the booze.

I pulled in, placed my order, got back on the road. Home was just a few minutes away.

Bed. Sleep. Forgetting. I would do that. And then...

That fucking truck.

Crash.

Everything went white. Then, black. I blinked. Or at least, I thought I did.

Where the fuck was I?

What the fuck just happened?

My ears rang. Metal groaned somewhere behind me, that awful, twisted sound cars make when they've been crushed into things they shouldn't have. I could smell oil. Gasoline. Burnt rubber. I reached up and felt something wet. Blood pouring from my right eye or where my right eye used to be.

Oh my God. Did I still have it? I couldn't tell.

I shoved the car door open and stumbled out. The air was cold, alive with sirens. Red and blue lights flickered off the wet asphalt like some kind of sick disco.

"What the fuck..." I muttered, spinning, dizzy. "What the fuck did I just do?"

Bits came back to me. The Dallas Country Club. The drinks. Tom's house. His mom's whisper. The party. The laughter. The beer. Those stupid fuckers pressing drinks into my hand like they were doing me a favor.

And me, I found myself smiling, taking them all. Never saying no. Never being able to say no. And now, this.

"My eye! My eye!" I screamed. "I lost my fucking eye!"

Someone shouted back, calm, almost bored, "Sir, you cut your eyelid. You're going to be okay."

The paramedics were on me then, hands, voices, lights. Everything blurry, it felt surreal. That's when it hit me.

I could've killed someone. Maybe I had. I didn't know. Didn't want to know.

I later heard it was a five or six-car pileup. I caused it. But I never looked it up. Couldn't bring myself to. All I knew was, I'd messed up, big time. Smashed my face, tore up my car, nearly lost an eye. But not my life. Somehow, I still had that.

When I woke up in the ER, I felt like I'd been dropped from the sky. Everything ached. There was a nurse beside me, whispering, "The police were here," she said softly. "You ought to be glad they didn't get your blood alcohol content."

She said a number, I don't remember it exactly, but it was high. Really, *really* high. Like, shouldn't-even-be-alive high. And yet, there I was. Breathing.

Gloria looked at me, quiet for a beat. "And you still didn't stop drinking," she said finally.

I laughed, a dry, bitter sound. "Nope. Not a snowball's chance in hell. Started seeing a counselor, though. Started moderating."

Her eyebrow arched. "And clearly, that worked out pretty well, didn't it?"

Damn. She was a Jersey girl.

126

Chapter Ten

I was dreaming peacefully, carving fickle narratives in my head. Should I talk to the client or not? What would come of it anyway? Was it even in the client's best interest? Just as I was about to get to the good part, the alarm blasted in my ear. Jesus. What a way to wake up.

I muttered to myself, *Well, that job's gone anyway. Sucked to begin with.*

Time for the morning routine. Prayer, prayer, prayer, and meditation.

I said three prayers every morning, without fail.

The Third Step Prayer.

The Seventh Step Prayer.

The Prayer of St. Francis.

And then, of course, the Our Father, can't forget the Our Father.

I'd memorized all of them, which, honestly, I was pretty proud of. Not too many people could say that, huh? Then it was the daily devotions, gratitude list, text a few folks from the program, and meditate for twelve minutes. You'd think it'd be calming, but half the time it made me crazy. Like that old joke, "Don't mess with my freaking meditation!" I made that one up myself. Usually got a laugh or two. I thought I was pretty damn clever.

Quick breakfast. Protein shake. God, these freakin' diets sucked. But whatever, I had to keep the gut down. Then off to the gym. Quick 30 minutes on the treadmill with the TV going in the background. That helped. As long as it wasn't CNN. I couldn't stand CNN or their circus of talking heads.

Back home. Quick change. No time for a shower. Straight to the meeting. A speaker night, followed by fellowship and dinner at Saltgrass. One of our buddies had just picked up his three-year chip. Another guy, same name, thirty-two years sober. Go figure.

The steak was heaven. Juicy. Every bite was worth the calories. I even had a little bread. A cheat. Screw it. I hated this damn diet anyway. Went back home, did some small talk, then bed.

Next morning, new day. Rushed again. I'd found a new church. Maybe this was the one that would finally save my soul for good. How many times had I said that before? Too many. But apparently not enough. I knelt on the floor, cried a little, prayed hard, then had my coffee, which was sweet, strong, black. My one non-negotiable. They could take my vodka, but not my coffee. Not yet.

Then I met this girl. Dominique. From Houston. Cute as hell. Bright eyes, voice like silk. I thought maybe she was the one. But of course, she had a boyfriend. We talked for a few minutes, shared a laugh, I got some more coffee, and left. Rush, rush, rush. Always rushing.

I had to meet Roxy; we were checking out this new meeting for people who'd grown up in total chaos. Adult Children of Alcoholics and Other Dysfunction. ACA. Sounded like my tribe.

Traffic was a nightmare. God, I hated Dallas traffic. Still trying to learn my way around, and now I was stuck at the damn interchange when Roxy called. Shit, there were no hands-free in this rental, and my damn car was still in the shop after the wreck.

I picked up anyway. "Hey, Roxy, I'm on the way…" But she'd already hung up. Traffic, traffic, rush, rush, rush. Finally, I made it. Then the phone rang again. "I thought you were gonna let me know when the meeting was," Roxy said.

"Oh, I'm sorry," I told her. "It's been chaos, but here's where it is. I'll wait for you." She showed up, big smile, big hug, kiss on the cheek. That's how besties roll, and then the discussion started, another meeting, another room, another story.

I shared my heart that night, like I usually did. Maybe a little over the top, but well, that's me. What's the point of holding back, right?

When the meeting wrapped up, they did that thing, called for newcomers, and asked if anyone wanted to take a desire chip. Just like in AA. And Roxy, damn, she surprised me. She raised her hand, walked up, and asked for a chip and a newcomer's packet. She'd taken the leap.

Right then, I knew, we were in this together. As we walked out, we stopped to look over the ravine below the building. "Such a pretty view," Roxy said. "I'd like to go out and see that."

Funny thing, I'd been there plenty of times and never noticed how deep and green it really was. Guess I wasn't looking close enough. She saw it right away. And then I saw the steps. Oh, shit. I hated steps. Freaking multiple sclerosis.

"It's okay," she said, reading my mind. "I got you."

So I took the leap, literally and figuratively. I put my trust in her, gave her my vote of confidence, and started down. After a few shaky steps, she turned around, looked at me, and said,

"Here, hold onto my shoulders. I'll guide you down. I won't let you fall."

And so, I did. I followed her carefully, hands resting on her shoulders, step by step, scared shitless the whole way. My legs were trembling. My heart was pounding, but I didn't fall. When we got to the bottom, she said softly, "Let's stop here."

We stood there, looking out over the ravine. The green, the stillness, the peace, it all hit me at once. I could finally breathe.

"Can I hug you?" I asked.

"Yeah," she said, and I did.

Then she looked right at me, eyes honest and steady. "You know, thinking about that meeting, there was so much that went on in my family. So many lies. So much swept under the rug. It's not like AA. I get what you meant now. I couldn't have done this earlier. Good thing I waited eighteen months. It means so much that you invited me."

"Thanks," I said. "It was the same for me. I got sober in January 2016, but I didn't start this program again until September 2017. Tried it before in 2010. Didn't work. Doesn't really work when you're not sober."

"I get it," she said. "No way I could've done this back then either. I like this meeting, though. I'm gonna keep coming."

She paused for a moment, then looked at me again. "You know, Tad, I understand you more and more. And the more I do, the more I think it's no accident we met. We met exactly when we were supposed to. You're strong, and brave, and kind. You say you're not, but you are. What you've been through, most people would've turned into assholes. But not you. You're still loving. You're still trying." I blinked, not sure what to do with that. She kept going. "You're strong, you're brave, you're intelligent, you're handsome, and you're so, *so* stubborn."

I raised an eyebrow at her.

She laughed. "You are. But you had to be. That's what kept you alive. I'm lucky to have you as a friend. And I don't say that to many people. You're one of the few."

I smiled. I didn't really know if that's what real friends did, say things like that, but I'd take it. Roxy was my friend. One I'd do anything for. I loved her to the moon and back.

"Come on, Tad," she said, grinning. "Let's go to dinner. You can meet the kitties. I'll help you up. Grab my hand." And I willingly did.

******

The day started out... well, normally. Which for me means *blah*. That's my default setting, waking up hating the world, everyone in it, and everything about it. Only the comfort of my old sofa blanket, a little prayer and meditation, and a good, strong cup of coffee could ever soften the edge. That's where I was this morning, grumpy, sluggish, but functioning.

Didn't have much on the agenda. A few errands. Some time at the gym. Then later, I was supposed to meet up with friends to watch the debate between Ted Cruz and Colin Allred. Easy enough. Everything was going fine until I called the damn doctor's office.

There was some issue with coverage for my MS meds. Again. There's *always* an issue. The old me would've lost it, would have screamed, cursed, slammed the phone against the wall, but I've had years of therapy and step work now. Supposedly, I'm better at this "staying calm" thing.

So, I took a breath and I tried to reason.

I told the receptionist, "You know, the *old me* wouldn't be so nice. In fact, I'm actually shouting a million expletives at you in my head right now, but I still need your help. If this were a survey, and one was terrible and five was perfect, I'd give you a '1' and that's me being generous, okay?" There was a pause. I could feel the rage pulsing under my skin, but I held it down. "What's your name?" I asked.

"Naomi," she said.

"Okay, Naomi," I said, doing my best to sound human, "here's the deal. You said I could leave my name and number, and somebody would call me back, but they never do. So I'm gonna wait right here on the phone until I can talk to someone. I'd hate to have to get lawyers involved."

That got her attention. She said she'd "be right back."

And I waited. Forever. I'd finished my coffee by the time she came back on, but at least the hold music was classical. I love classical. It's the one thing that keeps me from completely losing my shit.

Finally, Naomi came back. "Okay, Mr. Jaehrling, they're going to have to call you back. Will you please give me a number, and they'll call you right back?"

Of course.

Of course.

I hung up. Muttered a few choice words. Then went on with my errands.

By the time I got home, the phone rang again, it was my brother. Normally, I'd let it go to voicemail, but we've had a rocky relationship since my meltdown, and I figured maybe I should try to be better. We ended up talking for an hour. It was actually good. Healing, even. Maybe we were finally finding our footing again after Mom's passing and the whole mess with her accounts. For a moment, it felt like progress.

And then, as usual, the universe said, "Not so fast."

The nurse from the doctor's office called with her obnoxiously sweet voice. Told me I'd be getting an email to complete my application for hardship assistance. Fine.

When I got home from the gym, there it was, the email with the form. I opened it, or tried to. It took *forever*. The thing looked like it was designed by a committee of sadists. Still, I tried. Clicked every link, refreshed the page, and cursed under my breath. Then it froze. Wouldn't open. Wouldn't move. That's when I lost it.

I screamed. Loud. Full-throated, red-faced, vein-popping scream. I cursed God in every language I knew, and a few I probably made up on the spot. And then I just sat there, breathing hard, staring at the screen, thinking, *Here we go again.* The same damn cycle. The chaos that, no matter how hard I try, never seems to let me go.

There was no two ways about it, MS sucked. As I always say, "I wouldn't recommend it." That's been my go-to line, my dry attempt at humor to make peace with something I never asked for and still resent on most days. I remember thinking, *why me?* Of all people, why did it have to be me? But life doesn't take requests, and I didn't get a choice.

So, after moving to Dallas, I decided to do what I've always done when something threatens to pull me under, I got proactive. I started looking for the best MS specialist I could find and eventually landed on a physician. One of the reasons I was so damn insistent was because I could feel it, I was slipping. My mind, the thing I'd always relied on, wasn't firing quite the same way.

People used to tell me, "My gosh, Tad, your memory amazes me!" And they weren't wrong. My memory had been my secret weapon. It's how I survived school, aside from the endless middle and elementary school bullying that came with it. I was the kid whose lunch got thrown across the schoolyard just for sport.

I remember one day, we were in class, and a flock of birds landed outside on the lawn. The teacher looked out the window and said, "What's going on out there?" Some kid snorted, "Oh, that's Tad's lunch." A few laughs followed. I was the joke of the day again. It's no wonder I grew up miserable. No wonder I trashed every single yearbook later on.

That was Josephina's idea, in a way. My partner at the time had this brilliant suggestion that I should "declutter." I wasn't even a clutterer, but she liked to control things. So, I figured, *fine, kill two birds with one stone.* Avoid a fight and get rid of the ghosts from Piney Woods Christian Academy. Into the shredder they went. Goodbye, PWCA. You're dead to me. Well, except for a couple of classmates, I still keep in touch with. The irony.

The thing is, having a memory like mine has always been both a blessing and a curse. It helped me blaze through school, even when life threw distractions my way. Eventually, I pulled it together, earned my MBA from Rice, became a certified analyst, and made something of myself. Pretty good for a guy who was told he'd succeed *if* he could just "learn how to deal with people better." Not exactly a skill my parents excelled at teaching.

I've made my own way, and for the most part, it's worked. But I've always been hyper-aware of my mind, how sharp it feels, how quickly it catches things. Especially now, after watching what's been happening to my mom. It scared me enough to start taking memory tests just to be sure I was still me. Then I saw something I never thought I'd see in a million years: my scores slipping. Not by much, but enough for me to notice. And I wasn't having it. So, I went looking for answers.

One neurologist in Plano didn't sugarcoat it. I brought in the brain scans, and he looked them over, then said, matter-of-factly, "Yep, you do have MS."

"Thanks. That's good news," I said, in my usual dry tone.

He smirked a little and said, "But I can tell you're smart."

"Oh really? How so?" I asked.

"The eyes," he said. "You're alert. You're aware."

I didn't know what to say to that, but I appreciated it. He referred me to a neurologist, and that's where things finally started making sense. The new doc was different, sharp, personable, and, most importantly, he actually listened to me.

When we sat down, I showed him everything, the scans, the test results, the little dips in my memory that felt like cracks in a foundation I'd spent decades building.

"What am I going to do?" I told him. "My mind is everything to me. If I lose that, I'm sunk."

He leaned back, calm as ever, and said, "Well, I think we have a solution." Then he started telling me about this new drug called Tysabri.

The thing about Tysabri was, it sounded no less than a miracle drug. Administered by injection, it was supposed to help

135

people with MS radically improve both their physical health and mental sharpness. My doctor was convinced it could work for me. "Only catch," he said, "you'll need to get tested for something called the John Cunningham Virus… JCV."

Apparently, if you had JCV, the drug could backfire spectacularly after about a year, causing long-term brain damage and possibly severe cognitive decline. Great. Exactly what I needed, right? But still, it was worth a shot.

He looked at me, waiting for my answer. "Are you willing to take the chance?" he asked.

"Heck yeah," I said without hesitation. What did I have to lose?

We made the arrangements right then and there. I'd get tested for the virus, and if the results came back clean, I'd have a real shot at keeping my brain intact, maybe even for the rest of my life. And honestly, taking risks was nothing new for me. I'd driven cross-country once to try my hand at acting in Hollywood. I'd gotten LASIK surgery back when it was still practically an experiment because I was tired of squinting at the world through Coke-bottle lenses. I'd taken a ten-thousand-dollar inheritance from my grandmother and used it to start a real estate business. I'd even turned down a steady job as a portfolio manager to buy a tanning salon franchise in League City. Yeah, I wasn't exactly allergic to risk. So, taking a gamble on Tysabri? That was nothing.

Immediately after the appointment, I went straight to get tested for JCV. Two weeks later, a rep from the drug manufacturer called to schedule my first injection. It took them a while to find a spot that could fit me in; apparently, people lined up for this stuff, but they finally landed on a clinic off Central Expressway that did the treatments on Saturdays. "Perfect," I told them.

The following weekend, I was actually excited, something I hadn't felt in a while. I stopped by a sandwich shop, grabbed a chicken sandwich, chips, and a drink, and then headed over. I checked in, went through the usual paperwork routine, and soon they called me back to the treatment room.

It was a big, bright room lined with recliners where patients sat hooked up to their IVs. The place had this odd, clinical coziness to it. There were snacks everywhere, coffee (which instantly lifted my mood), M&Ms, mini Snickers, and Goldfish crackers. You name it. I was told to plan for about two hours, so I settled in for the long haul.

I grabbed a bottle of water, loaded up on snacks like a kid at recess, and made myself a coffee with French Vanilla creamer. Then I picked a big white recliner by the window, figured I might as well have a view while someone pumped medication into me.

The staff was friendly and efficient, which helped. My nurse, Carla, came over to take my vitals, temperature, and blood pressure, and then started prepping the IV. She was quick. Watching her, I couldn't help myself, and I told her something.

"You do that pretty well," I said.

She smiled. That was all the invitation I needed. Conversation was my default setting. I learned she'd just moved from Mississippi and missed her family, but was starting to like Dallas. I asked about her weekend plans, what she liked to do for fun, and what she had going on for Easter.

Why not? Talking was what I did best. I spent my career asking people about their families, their hobbies, and their thoughts on the stock market, then offering a little expert guidance, of course. I was the analyst, after all.

Eventually, the talk drifted to politics, my favorite rabbit hole. I couldn't resist. My uncle had been in the business, so I always figured I had the inside scoop, the "right answers." Not everyone agreed, of course, but they were too polite to say so. That was the beauty of it, people would nod along, pretend to be engaged, and I'd get to keep holding court. And honestly, I did have good judgment. Most of the time.

So, there I was, sitting in that big white chair, IV in my arm, sipping coffee, eating Goldfish, talking about the world like I had it all figured out, while my brain, somewhere in the background, quietly prayed this drug would give me a fighting chance to stay myself.

After I finished eating, I pulled out my phone to see what kind of madness the world was serving up that day. Sure enough, the war in Ukraine was still burning, and politicians were still screaming about the border. Same song, different verse.

I could almost hear my dad, Al Jaehrling, in the back of my head saying what he always used to say, "It never stops. All my life, we've always been at war in some way or another. Will we ever have peace?" Evidently not. So, the mayhem rolled on, just in headlines instead of artillery fire.

Carla came back over, checked my pulse and blood pressure again, and asked which arm I wanted to use. "Left," I told her. She nodded, prepped the solution, wiped my arm with an alcohol swab, and slid the needle into that big vein running down my left arm. The sting was quick, and then the IV started its slow drip. I watched the clear fluid make its lazy way down the tube, wondering if that was what hope looked like, cold, sterile, and hanging from a steel stand.

While the medicine did its thing, I went back to doing what I did best, talking. Politics, culture, finance, you name it. I was in full swing, preaching to my tiny audience of nurses and assistants, most of whom were either pretending to care or silently plotting my death. Hard to tell which. But that didn't matter. I kept going. Somebody had to save the world, right? By 4:30, it was all done. Carla came over, tapped the machine, ran through the post-checks, made sure every last drop had gone in, and unhooked me.

And that was that. The ordeal was over, though honestly, it hadn't been bad at all. Truth be told, I kind of liked the attention, people fluttering around me, checking vitals, making sure I was okay. For once, I was the center of someone's universe, even if it was just for a couple of hours and mostly because I was hooked up to a bag of chemicals.

A week later, I went in for my follow-up with the neurologist. I was feeling great, optimistic even. I couldn't wait to tell him how smooth the first treatment had gone. I raved about the staff, the snacks, and the whole setup. And most of all, how relieved I was that I didn't have the John Cunningham Virus. That meant I could stay on Tysabri for life, keep my brain sharp, my body steady. Then I noticed the doctor giving me a heavy stare that lasted just a little too long.

"You do have the virus," he said.

And just like that, the bottom fell out.

Chapter Eleven

You ever have one of those days where you feel like a sack of wet cement being dragged through your own life? That was me. Between the insurance fiasco, the new meds, and the general existential dread that came with MS, I was about ready to throw in the towel and spend the entire day watching reruns of *The Office* with a bag of Goldfish and a pity blanket. But something in me, it wasn't motivation, let's be honest, more like guilt or stubbornness, said, *Go, Tad. Just show up.*

So I did.

The room was, as always, warm, and smelled faintly of coffee and peppermint. Folding chairs in a circle, fluorescent lights humming above, the usual assortment of wounded-but-functional souls. I took a seat near the back, my standard spot. Safe. Unassuming. Close enough to bolt if I got sick of myself halfway through. That's when I noticed her.

She was sitting across the circle, blonde hair pulled into a low ponytail, a soft gray sweater that looked like it had survived both a thrift store and a heartbreak. She wasn't talking, just listening, nodding occasionally, but there was something in her stillness, something steady, like she'd built a house in the middle of her own storm and was just sitting there on the porch, watching the rest of us flail.

When it came time for me to share, I narrated the usual and earned the usual polite chuckles. Then I talked, too much, as usual, about how the world was exhausting, how I hated having to depend on anyone, how I couldn't tell if I was healing or just tired of my own drama. You know, I had to sprinkle somewhere in there some honesty or harshness of life as well.

I wasn't in a good mood, so I actually didn't care if I said too much. When I looked up, Claire was watching me, not pitying, not amused, just *seeing* me. And it threw me off.

After the meeting, I was halfway out the door when she caught up to me. "You have a real way with words," she said.

I laughed. "That's one way to say *talks too much*."

She smiled with a half-smirk that said she'd heard that joke before. "No, I mean it. You're brutally honest. Most people try to make their pain sound poetic. You just say it like it is."

"Yeah, well," I shrugged. "The poetry's been beaten out of me by life and insurance claims."

She laughed then. It was actually really beautiful. Alive in a way. We walked out to the parking lot together, that weird post-meeting quiet sitting between us. I was about to say something self-deprecating just to fill the space, but she beat me to it.

"You know," she said, "you're not wrong about being cynical. But sometimes cynicism is just disappointment wearing armor."

I stopped mid-step. "That's... oddly insightful for someone I just met."

She grinned. "I read a lot of Brene Brown."

I snorted. "That explains it. You're one of *those* people, emotionally intelligent and annoyingly self-aware."

"Guilty," she said. "But I wasn't always."

Turns out, Claire was a newcomer. She'd just started coming to ACA, trying to untangle the mess her alcoholic father left in her head. She told me she'd spent years pretending she was fine, smiling through therapy, overachieving at work, dating men she had to fix just to feel useful. I nodded like I didn't relate, but my stomach knew better.

We stood by our cars for almost an hour, talking about many things, I mean one thing led to another and the topics weren't boring, so we kept it in flow. Her voice had this calm cadence that made me forget how much pain she must've carried underneath it. I didn't flirt, couldn't. There was no energy for pretense. It was just two people too tired to lie anymore.

Before she left, she said, "I'll see you next week?"

And for some reason, I said, "Yeah, I'll be here." And I meant it.

Driving home, I caught myself smiling. Not the performative, "I'm fine" smile I'd practiced for years. The small, quiet kind that sneaks up when you feel seen. The smile I smile when Roxy is around, I should introduce her to Claire.

There was something in her eyes, the way she looked at you. It wanted me to tell her everything about myself, good and bad collided, which was strange. I didn't like sharing much with people, and strangers to be exact. But I wanted to tell her.

We'll see. She seems oddly nice.

Chapter Twelve

"What do you have to report today?" Tyler Dykisma peered over his glasses, those sharp, probing eyes cutting through the conference room's recycled air.

I cleared my throat. "Well, I'm working on the Johnson and Smith cases this week. You mentioned a couple others coming my way, right?"

Tyler nodded with exaggerated gravity. "Yeah, but let's get these finished first. Then I'll give you the next one."

"Got it," I said, already half tuned out.

He moved on, calling out names in that clipped tone of his. Steven. Diedra. Alexis. Johnson. One by one, they gave their updates, the same dull chorus of productivity and forced optimism. It was corporate theatre, the kind where no one cared about the performance, yet everyone had to applaud. I stared at the table, my mind drifting. The coffee in front of me had gone cold hours ago, and the fluorescent light above flickered just enough to make me wonder if it was trying to kill me. Finally, mercifully, the meeting ended.

Back at my desk, I downed what was left of the bitter coffee, tossed the paper cup in the trash, and went down the hall to the restroom, a ritualistic escape, if nothing else. When I came back, there was a handwritten note from Tyler sitting on my desk.

"Please do some research on Chevron for a client."

Now, this was the part of my job I actually liked. Research. Numbers. Patterns. Logic that didn't talk back.

Once upon a time, I wanted to be a full-fledged research analyst. But life, as usual, got creative with my plans. I'd taken a detour into entrepreneurship, a tanning salon that wanted to be a spa. It sounded more glamorous than it was. Machines instead of masseuses. Spray tans instead of serenity. It didn't exactly scream "professional growth." And yet, here I was, trying to claw my way back, working at a lower level than the job I'd once turned down to buy that damn salon. The irony wasn't lost on me.

Chevron looked good on paper: stronger fundamentals than its peers, solid cash flow, stable dividends. I put together a clean, polished analysis, added a few flourishes for Tyler's benefit, and sent it off. When I looked at the clock again, it was 7:00 p.m.

"Damn," I muttered. I'd forgotten how much the corporate world demanded from you, the hours, the grind, the illusion of upward motion. I packed up and bolted. Down the elevator. Out of the glass doors. Into my non-descript SUV. Traffic was hell as always. South Houston to downtown felt like an eternity. The roads were lined with brake lights stretching to infinity, each one pulsing red like a heartbeat. I turned on the radio. Christian music. The kind I used to listen to when I still believed God was listening back.

After thirty-five minutes, I pulled into the driveway of my little bungalow. It wasn't fancy, but it was mine. Snow and Ophelia, my two cats, were waiting like they owned the place. Snow was perched on the counter again. I yelled halfheartedly, and she jumped down, tail flicking like I was the one misbehaving.

Dinner was frozen pizza. Not the healthiest option, but at that point in my life, nutrition felt more like an optional lifestyle choice. I preheated the oven, set the timer for eighteen minutes, and told myself I'd atone at the gym tomorrow. When the timer beeped, I ate at the counter, phone in hand, doomscrolling through headlines I'd already read three times that week. War. Politics. Outrage. Repeat.

The next morning, I walked into the office and braced for Tyler.

He stood at the head of the conference table, already mid-lecture. "So, Dylan, tell us, how are your prospects looking? Have you continued making your calls?" Dylan answered on cue, full of forced confidence. Tyler nodded smugly, like a man pleased with his reflection.

I watched him, the bald spot glistening under the LED light, the intensity in his eyes almost theatrical. There was a cruelty in him, subtle but constant.

This guy, I thought. *What is he even talking about?*

Tyler droned on, then pivoted. "Now, let's talk about the Christmas party."

Marisa interrupted, "And it's no 'holiday party,' right?"

"You're darned right," Tyler snapped. "NO holiday parties here. Only Christmas parties. We only celebrate Christmas here."

He looked at me. "And Tad, you're coming early to help park the clients' cars."

I blinked. "Okay."

"Dylan, you and your wife come early to set up."

"Yes, sir!" Dylan said, overly enthusiastic.

"Now," Tyler continued, "let's talk wardrobe. Dylan and Charlene, jacket and a dress."

145

Dylan smirked. "You want me to wear the dress?"

"NO," Tyler barked. "You wear the jacket, she wears the dress." Someone, I don't remember who, asked, "What are you wearing, Tyler?"

"I might have to wear heels," he shot back. The room went dead quiet. No one breathed.

"The point being that I'm short," he added stiffly.

"You got it, boss," Dylan said quickly, rescuing us from implosion.

When the meeting ended, I was back at my desk, working on a plan for a new client, a recently widowed sixty-five-year-old woman with $1.5 million in assets and $90,000 in annual expenses. The numbers weren't promising. Six percent withdrawal rate. Not sustainable. But if she cut back to seventy thousand a year, she could probably make it to ninety-five without running out. Maybe even die richer than she lived. It was strange, advising people on how to live better with their money when I wasn't even sure I was living well with mine.

My phone buzzed. Sally. A friend from church. "Bible study tonight. You coming?" I looked at the clock, 5:25. Close enough to quitting time. I shut down my computer, grabbed my coat, and walked out. Before leaving, I turned back toward the office, the flickering light, the quiet hum of the computers, the faint smell of burnt coffee in the air.

For a second, I wondered how long I could keep playing this part, the diligent employee, the responsible adult, the man holding it all together. Then I exhaled, turned off the lights, and stepped into the hallway.

Tomorrow, it would all start again.

I was the last one to leave. Funny how that became a pattern in my life, being the last one standing in rooms I didn't even want to be in.

The year had been brutal. After I sold my tanning salon, my not-quite-spa with machines that hummed louder than the customers, I bounced into a job with a Turkish steel company that may or may not have been selling corroded steel to clients. That gig ended fast. Turns out, being part of a potential scandal isn't the best résumé bullet.

So, I did what people do when they're desperate and smart enough to admit it, I went to a state agency that helps people with disabilities find work. Depression and anxiety qualified me for the "mental health" category. They called it "vocational rehab." I called it survival.

That's how I met *him*.

Tyler Dykisma.

We met in person one afternoon, his desk spotless, his tie a shade too confident for a man his height. We talked a while. I watched the way he looked at me. I knew the game. So, I did what I'd been trained to do in sales, in business, in life: I closed him.

"I want this job," I said, leaning forward. "What's the next step?"

He paused, grinning like he'd just found a dollar bill on the sidewalk. "I'm tired of looking," he said. And that was that. A few days later, the offer came, $52,000 a year, no insurance. ACA coverage would have to do. Not much, but it was a paycheck. It meant I could keep my house, keep my cats, and maybe a chunk of my sanity. Tyler handed me a printed sheet when I signed the paperwork. In bold letters at the top, it read: Faith, Family, and Fun.

I wanted to laugh. But instead, I smiled and shook his hand.

Monday dawned cold and gray, the kind of rare Houston chill that seeps into your bones and your mood. I went through my routine: anxiety meds, shower, shave, dress, drive.

On the way, I called Dento, my friend, my occasional sponsor, and sometimes my sanity check. "Man, I don't know if I can do this job," I told him. "I feel like I'm walking into a firing squad every day."

"You just gotta get through it, brother," he said in his deep, easy voice. "You've done harder things." Maybe I had.

When I got to the office, I climbed the four flights of stairs to the fifth floor, pulled out my keys, and unlocked the door. First one there, as usual. The office was still, dark except for the glow from the EXIT sign. I sat down, turned on my computer, and let the silence stretch. I'd worked hard for years. People said I was talented, even brilliant, but somehow, I always got sideways with management.

Why was that? I knew I could be unpredictable. Sometimes timid and eager to please, other times harsh and explosive. I told myself it was passion, but the truth? It scared people.

There were the highlights or lowlights, depending on who you asked. The time I yelled at a temp because he couldn't balance a spreadsheet. The time I threw a highlighter that ricocheted off a doorframe and barely missed someone's head, or the day I told an employee with warts on his hands to "get those things burned off."

Not exactly leadership material.

And then there was *the big one*. The investment firm. The day the Chief Investment Officer said, "Management only for this meeting." I went anyway. And, of course, I spoke up. Loudly.

By the following week, I was packing my desk. I had a talent for blowing things up, especially when I started to feel invisible. So yeah, now I was here, under Tyler Dykisma, the human embodiment of a migraine. I was supposed to survive this? The odds weren't great.

When I first started, I told my dad, "Tyler's a good guy."

That was based on one photograph on his desk, him holding a baby, eyebrows raised in what I thought was innocence. That's how naïve I was. Tyler loved to talk about his "hard childhood." His mom was a teacher, apparently the gravest of hardships. The real red flag came later.

He told me, proudly, that he'd sold his Apple stock after Tim Cook came out as gay. "I don't think companies should be making those kinds of political statements," he said.

That one sat with me. The bigotry. The smugness. The financial stupidity. He sold Apple, one of the best-performing stocks of the decade, because the CEO was gay. Then he bought Twitter, right before it tanked. That's when I knew: Tyler wasn't just an asshole. He was a *dumb* asshole.

Weeks rolled by. The job was monotonous, the pay barely tolerable, but it was something to do. Something to wake up for. Then came *the Christmas picture*.

Tyler insisted it be taken late in the evening, long after normal office hours, of course. He wanted "dedication" in the frame.

His mother, Beersheba, was there too. She worked for him. Don't ask me why. Maybe she couldn't say no to her little prince. Maybe she thought enabling him was love.

149

Tyler was in rare form that night, smug, sweaty, self-satisfied. As we gathered for the picture, I heard him bark, "Look at this! Beersheba looks like a crack addict!" The room froze. No one spoke.

Even my own mom would have slapped me into next week if I'd ever talked to her like that. But Beersheba just stood there, silent, eyes down, her face the color of resignation. My heart broke for her. And then I understood. This little tyrant had been raised to believe cruelty was a form of strength. That he could humiliate people, even his own mother, and still call himself a man.

They say people like that are compensating for something. Tyler was five-foot-five, balding, beady-eyed, and overcompensating like it was a full-time job. We took the photos. A thousand of them. By the time we were done, it was almost 8 p.m. The rest of the team shuffled out, exhausted and tight-lipped. Tyler lingered. I lingered longer.

When I finally stepped into the elevator, the doors closed in front of me with a metallic sigh. My reflection stared back in the dull stainless steel. Tired eyes. Cracked optimism. A man trying to prove something no one was asking for.

Faith. Family. Fun.

That's what the paper had said.

I laughed under my breath.

"Yeah," I whispered. "Sure thing."

And the elevator hummed quietly down into the dark.

I got home and didn't even bother turning on the main light, just that little lamp by the sofa, the one that made everything look sepia and lonely. Snow was already on the counter, licking something invisible off the edge, and Ophelia gave me that slow, judgmental blink cats are born knowing how to do. I dropped my stuff on the floor. The sound felt too loud for how quiet the house was.

Most nights, I'd scroll through my phone or stare at the TV just to drown out the noise in my head, but tonight even that felt pointless. I just sat there. Hands folded. Staring. You know that kind of silence that's so thick you can hear your own heartbeat in your ears? That's what it was. My life had somehow shrunk to this tiny loop: work, traffic, reheated dinner, anxiety meds, and trying not to think about how everything I'd once been proud of had evaporated into nothing.

I rubbed my face hard. I felt used up. Like an old sponge. I glanced at my phone again. The screen lit up and I saw her name. Claire. She'd told me once she didn't sleep much either. "Trauma keeps office hours," she'd said. I hadn't laughed then. But I remembered it now.

I hit call before I could talk myself out of it. "Hey," she answered after two rings. Voice calm, a little hoarse as if she'd been reading before bed.

"Hey." I exhaled. "Sorry. It's late."

"It's fine," she said. "You sound like you need it."

I huffed out a laugh. "Do I?"

"Mhm."

"I just…" I stopped. It's funny how you forget how to talk about what actually hurts. "It's been a long day."

"Tyler again?"

"Tyler always." I leaned back, staring at the ceiling. "You ever met someone who just... makes you feel smaller every time you talk to them? Like you start the conversation human and end it as a bug?"

"Yeah," she said quietly. "My father." That hit harder than I expected. I didn't know what to say to that, so I didn't.

"I think I'm just tired," I went on after a bit. "Tired of pretending I don't hate it all. The meetings, the fake smiles, the way everyone laughs at his stupid jokes. I sit there thinking, *what the hell happened to me?* I used to want to be someone."

"You still are someone," she said.

"Yeah, but not the kind I wanted to be." The line went quiet for a while, but not empty. She had this way of listening. Not filling the space with clichés or pep talks. Just being there.

"I keep wondering," I said, "if maybe this is it. Maybe I just peaked somewhere back there and didn't notice. Maybe life isn't about getting better. Maybe it's just about learning how to sit with the disappointment."

"I think," she said, "it's about learning not to let disappointment be the whole story." I let that sit. It sounded simple. It wasn't.

"I don't know how to do that," I said.

"You don't have to," she said. "Not tonight." Something loosened in me then. I didn't even realize I'd been holding my breath until I exhaled and felt my shoulders drop. We stayed on the phone like that for a while, talking about nothing, then about everything. Her voice got softer as the minutes passed, the way the air gets quiet before dawn.

"I'm glad you called," she said eventually.

"Yeah," I whispered. "Me too."

Snow curled up next to me, purring like she approved. I leaned my head back, closed my eyes. For once, the silence didn't hurt. Just before I drifted off, I heard her breathing on the other end, and it felt like maybe, for tonight, that was enough.

Chapter Thirteen

I followed Tyler down the hallway like a man being led to his own execution. You could always tell when something was coming, that subtle change in the air. The whole office had been quiet all morning, unusually so. Even the intern, Emily, hadn't made her usual chipper comments about coffee or her classes.

When he called my name, "Tad, can I see you for a minute?" I already knew what it was. My stomach dropped clean through the floor.

He led me into his office, or as I'd started calling it in my head, *the lair, the* crocodile's den. There were Christmas ornaments still hanging around, one shaped something like a snowman with glitter peeling off, mocking me with its fake cheer. Perry Griffin was there, too. Corporate cleanup man. I'd seen that guy enough times to know what his presence meant. HR didn't show up for 'chats.'

Emily sat on the couch, looking down at her phone. Poor kid didn't know where to put her eyes.

"Go ahead and take a seat," Tyler said, gesturing to the chair across from his desk. His tone was casual, the kind people use when they've already made up their mind and just want to get the dirty work over with. I sat. The leather creaked under me, and for some reason, that sound felt louder than anything else in the room.

Tyler leaned back in his chair, fingers steepled like a pastor about to deliver bad news in a holy tone. "Tad, I think you know why we're here."

I swallowed. "I've got a guess."

He nodded, pretending to appreciate my honesty. "We've reviewed the trades you made last week. The error was significant. It's not something we can just overlook." There it was. The hammer. I could feel the heat rise in my face.

"I told you the system was unreliable. I said that from day one…"

He cut me off. "This isn't about the system. This is about accountability."

Accountability. God, I hated that word. It always sounded noble coming from people who'd never once admitted their own mistakes.

"I was trying to fix it before it blew up," I said. "I wasn't hiding it."

Tyler gave me that fake sympathetic look, the same one he probably practiced in the mirror when he told clients bad news. "Intentions don't change the outcome, Tad."

Perry cleared his throat, monotone. "We're going to need your badge and building access card." I stared at them both, blinking. It was like watching a movie I'd already seen a dozen times. The dialogue didn't change; the ending never did. Just the faces.

Tyler kept talking, something about learning experiences, about 'not letting this define me.' I barely heard him. My mind was a carousel of noise: *you idiot, you knew this was coming, you did it again, you always do this.* When I finally stood up, my legs felt like they weren't mine. I handed over my badge. My hands were trembling, not from fear, exactly, but from this deep, gnawing mix of shame and fury that sat right behind my ribs.

I wanted to say something clever. Something that would leave a scar. Instead, I just said, "Merry Christmas, Tyler."

He flinched, just a tiny one, and I took that as my parting gift. Then I walked out.

The hallway looked different now, emptier somehow. I passed the fake tree we'd decorated, its lights still blinking like a heartbeat that didn't know it was attached to a corpse. By the time I got outside, the cold air hit me; it felt similar to a hand smacking me across the face, hard. I just stood there, staring at my car, trying to catch my breath. This wasn't my first fall, but God, it still hurt like the first time.

I sat behind the wheel and gripped it until my knuckles turned white. *You did it again, Tad.* The words rotated in my head. *You blew it. You always blow it.*

Maybe this was who I was, a man who kept tripping over his own damn feet, trying to walk straight in a world built on crooked lines. I started the car. Drove home in silence. Snow was waiting at the door when I got there. I didn't even turn the lights on. Just dropped my coat on the floor, sat on the couch, and laughed, this bitter, hollow laugh that came from somewhere too deep to control.

Then I stopped. And for reasons I still don't fully understand, I picked up my phone.

Claire's name stared back at me.

I didn't call her. Not yet.

I just sat there, thumb hovering over the screen, thinking about how many times a person could screw up before they stopped being worth saving. I could tell by the look on Tyler's face the second I walked in, the man was about to swing a wrecking ball. He folded his hands, leaned forward, and hit me with it.

"I've lost confidence in you."

That was the first bullet. The rest followed clean and methodical, as if he'd practiced them in the mirror. But why would he waste his efforts on me? He was just so used to pulling the rug from people's feet that it got smoother and smoother over time. When he hired me, he said he was *impressed* by my analyst background. *Impressed.* That word aged like milk. Now I was a mistake, another entry in his managerial cautionary tale.

He went through the list: missed trades, miscalculations, poor judgment calls. My own personal greatest hits. Each one stung, but the worst part was knowing he wasn't entirely wrong.

"So, it's time for us to part as friends." No severance. No reference. No help finding another gig. Just an HR guy in the corner pretending not to enjoy the show.

I managed to croak, "Okay… I'm going to file for unemployment."

Tyler barely blinked. "I'll fight it," he said. "I have lawyers."

Of course he did.

"I've got MS," I said, voice shaking now. "I have expenses. What am I going to live on?"

"You have assets."

And that was that. Conversation over. He stood up and offered his hand. I shook it. Why was it so goddamn sweaty?

How could I have been so stupid? I turned down an interview with a major bank for this smug son of a bitch. For what? A smaller title and a promise of "growth potential"?

I sat in my car, trying to decide between blasting the radio or just sitting in silence. Ended up doing both, silence first, then noise. Didn't help either way. Back home, my phone buzzed. A text from Tyler.

"Sorry that had to happen, Tad. I appreciated your hard work, but it just wasn't a good fit."

I stared at it until the letters blurred. *Not a good fit.* So I changed my Facebook religion from "Christian" to "spiritual." It was the least I could do. That night, I sat in the dark, staring at my Smith & Wesson. It wasn't about pulling the trigger. It was about how *comforting* it felt to hold something that could make the noise stop, if I ever wanted it to. Instead, I did everything except then and went on thinking and thinking as if my sanity depended on it. I went to bed. The cats needed food. The bills needed paying. Reality has a way of keeping you alive.

The next morning, I dragged myself to the men's group. Told them everything, the firing, the humiliation, the text. One guy, a self-proclaimed spiritual advisor, nodded gravely and said, "Man, you've got bad luck."

Bad luck. Right. Like it was weather. Like I just happened to walk under a leaky sky. That night, I did the math, $3,200 in liquid assets. Mortgage at $1,400 a month. Two months of breathing room, give or take. I had a tenant out back who paid $600. Enough to buy cat food and cheap coffee, not much else. I could pull from my IRA, but that meant taxes. My Roth? That meant guilt. So, I made a decision: I'd live on air, faith, and credit cards until the universe stopped kicking me in the teeth.

Dinner with friends came next, people I'd helped find an apartment once upon a time, when I was pretending to be a real estate agent. 7:30 dinner. I left the house at 7:30. The place was a wreck. I picked up clothes, took down the sad little Christmas tree, and told myself it was progress. It wasn't.

I arrived at 8:03. "Sorry, had a lot going on," I said. Understatement of the year.

We had Italian. Split a bottle of red. I couldn't afford it, but red wine was like an old lover; it burned going down, but it still made me feel something. Two glasses. My last, I told myself. I didn't believe it.

Sunday rolled in as sharp as my reality. I shuffled around the house, half-dressed, half-human. Tried to convince myself I was "looking for a job." Mostly, I just rearranged the wreckage. Rome was burning, and I was folding laundry. By afternoon, I knew I needed to *do* something. Anything.

I called up Dento, an old friend from AA.

"Yeah," he said. "Meet me at the clubhouse." He asked me how much I'd been drinking.

"Last week I had five on Saturday," I said. "And two glasses of wine last night." I left out the Saturday beers. What was the point?

"So that's it?" he said. "Five drinks one weekend and two glasses last night?"

"Yeah."

He nodded slowly. "Dude, I don't think alcohol is your problem. There's something else going on with you."

I looked at him. "What, then?"

He shrugged. "Try Al-Anon."

Perfect. Just perfect. Another room full of people who'd tell me to "let go and let God." But maybe he was right. Maybe I wasn't drinking to escape. Maybe I was drinking to *feel normal.*

To feel something normal. I don't know what normal is. At least, that I am sure of. It is this pedestal feeling that I keep searching for, and the way my life is unfolding, I don't think it actually exists, and my mind just likes obsessing over something far off in the distance because it somewhat promises a valid change. It promises a way out of misery. It keeps clinging onto this hopeful bird of a feeling, and I think, deep down, in my gut, I know it had gone extinct a long time ago.

But I like the chase.

Chapter Fourteen

I liked my job well enough. Friendly coworkers, decent clients, nice-enough management. It wasn't bad, it was just fine. The trouble was, fine doesn't pay the bills. I wasn't making the kind of money I thought I *should* be making. I'd check my account sometimes and feel my stomach twist, the kind of twist that made me vulnerable to scheisters with perfect smiles and 'game-changing opportunities.'

And sure enough, one found me.

A recruiter reached out on LinkedIn. Said she'd "been following my career trajectory." That made me laugh. There wasn't much of a trajectory to follow, unless you counted a series of sideways moves with occasional self-sabotage. But she talked a good game.

"You've got the perfect background," she said. "Credentialed, educated, experienced."

Hell, even I wanted to hire me after that.

The firm, some high-end financial outfit, had everything. The salary was double what I made. Full benefits. Paid vacation. A 401(k) match so generous it felt like divine intervention.

A gift from God, I thought. Except I should've remembered that God doesn't recruit through LinkedIn. Still, I got swept up in the flattery. The interviews started, and both sides wined and dined, well, metaphorically. They told me I was the best thing since sliced bread; I told them they were the end-all be-all of financial service firms. That's how this dance always went.

The lady in management compared it to dating. "Sometimes it works, sometimes it doesn't," she said with a shrug. Easy for her to say. She wasn't the one moving 250 miles away while her mom lost herself to dementia back home. But sure, let's call it dating.

I practiced for the interviews like a man auditioning for salvation. Spent hours in front of my laptop, rehearsing answers, perfecting smiles. I could practically hear the ghost of my old acting coach whispering, *"Less grimace, more gravitas."*

Then came the Big Interview, the one with the decision makers. If they liked me, I'd be packing for Dallas.

They asked the usual questions:

"How serious are you about being an analyst?"

"Have you ever worked at a major firm before?"

"Why did you leave the business?"

"What are you most proud of?"

"What did you do wrong?"

"Would your family be okay with you moving?"

And the kicker, "Would your mother be okay with it?"

I didn't know what to say to that.

Mom was… complicated. Bitter and brittle with age, but still my mom. We'd been close once, when I was younger, when life hadn't had so many edges. After I gave up on acting and moved back from California, I'd stayed with her for a while. That lasted about as long as a polite dinner.

When I landed that adhesive tape company job, running North American operations, she'd told me it was "high time I leave the nest." She found me an apartment locator, paid my deposit, and bought me a sofa bed.

That was Kitty Jaehrling, tough love wrapped in sarcasm. I didn't appreciate it then, but later I realized she'd done me a favor. Some people my age still lived at home. Kitty made sure I didn't become one of them.

After that, I never moved back. Not even when things with Francesca ended.

Ah, Francesca. Sensible, kind, patient, the kind of woman who'd hand you a towel instead of telling you you're an idiot for walking in the rain. She didn't like my ways, though. Not the restlessness, not the temper. Two and a half years, and then she was gone.

I asked her once if she'd take me back. She said, "No way, José." I laughed when she said it. Then I cried later, alone in the car. I think about her a lot, mostly when I start believing I've grown wiser. So there I was, packing my life into boxes, thinking Dallas might be my clean slate.

I drove into the city with that hopeful, itchy feeling you get before a new chapter, then saw the building. Big white corporate monolith. And on my phone, I caught a glimpse of the company's customer rating: *3.1 out of 5.*

Wait. What? Everyone had said this place was incredible. "Top-rated," "innovative," "family culture." If that were true, why did clients seem to hate it? That should've been my first red flag. But no, I was too busy feeling "chosen." Inside, I met my manager's manager, the HR team, some folks who all seemed one motivational quote away from collapsing. But no coworkers.

Turned out, there *were* no coworkers. I was the first hire for the Dallas division. My teammates? Scattered in another state. I met them over a glitchy video call where everyone smiled too wide. "Welcome to the team!" someone said. "You're gonna love it here."

I nodded. "Looking forward to it." And in that moment, I believed it.

Training started with endless modules, compliance tests, acronyms I'd never heard of. My clients were all overseas, which was a new flavor of loneliness. I missed handshakes, coffee meetings, real conversation. Everything here was screens and passwords. Then came the background check. They needed me to disclose "past incidents." That meant Waco. The "disagreement with some police officers" in the late '80s. I hesitated before writing it down. But I did it. Honesty, they said, was paramount. They liked to say "brutal honesty."

Funny thing, though, people love the idea of honesty until you actually give it to them. Still, I was happy. Happy as a clam, as they say. Making over a hundred grand, out of Houston, breathing fresh air again.

The firm felt like a second chance. A reward. Proof that God hadn't forgotten about me, even if I sometimes forgot about Him. Sure, all hell was breaking loose in Houston, Mama's dementia, my father's slow unraveling but here in Dallas, things were tranquil. I'd walk around the campus in early December, the red maple leaves falling like lazy confetti, and think, *Look at me. I made it.*

Finally, a man with a plan.

Finally, something stable.

Of course, the funny thing about stability is that it always looks solid until you press on it.

And I was about to press.

I started noticing the cracks about three months in. Tiny fissures at first, the kind you think you can live with, until one day the whole damn wall comes down. Why was everyone always so frantic?

Why did they move around like the building was on fire, and no one had told me?

People rushed the halls with phones glued to their ears, their eyes darting as if they were prey animals. Half of them talked so fast I was sure they'd crushed up Adderall into their morning coffee.

I knew they hadn't, but it sure looked that way. And everyone acted like what we were doing was divine work. Like the fate of the free world depended on a client's portfolio allocation in Luxembourg. It didn't. I knew it didn't. But saying that out loud would've made me the heretic of the bullpen.

And that's what it was, a bullpen. Rows and rows of pods, desks jammed together, the air thick with fluorescent buzz and panic. Phones ringing, people repeating the same script over and over. "Hi, Mr. So-and-so, just wanted to touch base about your account…"

"Hi, Ms. So-and-so, let's discuss your distribution options…" It was like living inside a broken record.

I remember asking one of my pod mates once, "Do you ever get tired of saying the same thing fifty times a day?"

He didn't even look up. "Follow the script, man. The script works."

"Oh," I said. "Right. Of course." Because heaven forbid we use originality, that might ruin the illusion of "personalized service." There was one guy, nice enough, who showed me how to set up a client distribution one day. He was kinda efficient and smart. Clearly miserable.

When we wrapped up, I checked my watch. "Lunch?"

He looked at me like I'd suggested we rob a bank. "Lunch? No time for lunch."

"You're kidding."

He shook his head. "Nope. Every now and then, I get to rest. Doesn't happen often. Enjoy this downtime while you have it." Then he stared at me with these flat, caffeine-stained eyes that said *this place will eat you alive if you let it.*

I didn't let it show, but my stomach sank a little.

Two months later, I was fully licensed and approved, officially a "Financial Advisor." The title looked good in email signatures. Clients started coming in, mostly high-net-worth types overseas.

Turned out, people in Singapore and people in Houston worried about the same thing: that they wouldn't outlive their money.

It was oddly comforting. Universal fear, I guess. Meanwhile, back home in Houston, things were falling apart. Mama was slipping deeper into dementia, and poor Emma, God bless her, was dealing with all of it.

Funny how I used to think she was over-emotional, always worked up about something. Turns out, she had every right to be. The woman was managing chaos with her bare hands while I was up here juggling spreadsheets. I respected her more than

166

I ever said out loud. She had this quiet strength I couldn't imitate, no matter how many self-help books I read. All that was happening while the world outside burned: politics, pandemics, pundits, panic. Everyone pretending to have the answers while barely keeping it together.

And me? I was falling apart in a different way. Quietly. Methodically. Like a professional.

The MS flared up when it wanted to, my hands sometimes shaking as I typed. The stress didn't help. Neither did the coffee, gallons of it. But coffee was the only vice left. I'd quit drinking five years ago. Quitting again wasn't an option. Meetings helped. Every Friday, every Saturday, I'd sit in those church basements and try to breathe. Try to remember I wasn't the only one spinning. But come Monday, it was back to the circus.

And then there was my mouth. I've always had one. Unfiltered, a relic from my father's fire-breathing temper and my mom's vodka-soaked honesty. Some people say, "Speak your truth."

I took that a little too literally.

Clients didn't love it. Apparently, "authentic" isn't what you want in a financial advisor. They complained. Management noticed. And one morning, after a year of trying to fit into this machine that never quite made space for me, I got an email.

Subject: "Quick chat. Video."

And that was how this specific hell, kicked me out. Didn't even bother with a face-to-face clash. Just a quick glitchy strike.

Chapter Fifteen

I should've shut up. God, how many times have I told myself that?

You'd think after forty-something years on this earth, a few burned bridges, and more than enough bruised egos to fill a therapy group, I'd learn the art of restraint. But no, not Tad Jaehrling. Nope. My mouth still had a mind of its own.

It happened on a Friday, always a damn Friday, when people were too tired to fight back but too awake to forget. I was on the phone with a client who'd been transferred to me, and he started spouting off some nonsense about 'the market being rigged by the global elite.' I mean, come on.

So, I asked the question that killed the deal, "Where exactly are you getting your news?"

He told me. And like an idiot, I told him why that was a terrible idea. Gave him a full-on sermon about responsible media consumption. By the end, I was basically the CNN of moral outrage, and he was staring at me through the phone line like I'd insulted his mother.

Monday morning, my manager pinged me. "Hey Tad, the client's being reassigned."

No preamble, no soft landing. Just that polite, corporate guillotine. And that was that.

I sat there staring at the email for a long while, that tight, acidic lump building in my throat again. I could almost hear Claire's voice in my head, *You know, not everything needs your correction.* She was right, damn it. But old habits die harder than old men.

Two days later, I received a call. It was that kind of early where the sun's still rubbing the sleep out of its eyes.

"Your Dad's gone," the person said, flat. At first, I thought they meant gone as in wandered off. That happened sometimes, his confusion taking the wheel, but no, it meant the actual *gone*. The gone with no return ticket. Heart attack. Collapsed in the kitchen. Bled out before the ambulance even showed. I don't remember hanging up. I just remember my keys hitting the counter, my body moving on autopilot, my brain gone to static.

Houston was gray when I landed. Or maybe it was just me. The house smelled like time had stopped. Old wood. Stale coffee. My mom's ghost lingering in every damn curtain. Emma was there, handling logistics, bless her frantic little heart. Claire showed up too, quiet, steady, like she'd been there a hundred times before. She didn't say much. Just handed me a bottle of water, put a hand on my shoulder, and started talking to the funeral director about floral arrangements. Shielding me from the cousins who wanted to "catch up."

God, I loved her for that.

When it came time for the eulogy, everyone turned toward me as if I was supposed to know what to say. I didn't, but I spoke anyway.

I said Dad was complicated. That he was tough on the outside, softer somewhere underneath. That he worked hard, maybe too hard. That he never really knew how to say what he felt, so he showed it by fixing things, paying bills, and keeping gas in our cars. And then, somewhere in the middle of that ramble, I looked at his casket and felt this weird thing happen inside me.

169

Forgiveness. Not the Hallmark kind, not clean or easy but the messy, reluctant kind that leaks out when you're too tired to hold the grudge anymore.

He was who he was, and so was I. And maybe that was enough.

I could almost see him there, shaking his head. "You're still talking too much, boy."

Yeah, Dad. Probably. It was unbearable while it lasted, probably added eighty percent of trauma into my cart, but... it wasn't truly bad having you around.

After the burial, people milled around the cemetery, whispering about casseroles and insurance. Claire stood beside me, hands tucked in her coat pockets, eyes down on the fresh dirt.

"You did good," she said quietly.

I laughed, a dry, broken sound. "Did I?"

She shrugged. "You showed up. Sometimes that's all that counts." We stood there for a long while, just listening to the wind moving through the trees. No need for speeches or fixes or prayers that didn't fit anymore. Just silence, the kind that finally didn't scare me.

I wasn't trying to run from the weight in my chest. I let it sit and somewhere between the graves and the gray sky, I swear I heard Al telling me it was okay to put it down.

Chapter Sixteen

I never really thought of myself as an entrepreneur. Hell, I barely thought of myself as employable most days, but I wanted to be one *badly*. I used to sit there for hours as a kid, flipping through *Forbes*, circling names on the "400 Richest Americans" list like they were baseball cards. Gates. Buffet. Walton. If only I could be one of them, I'd think. If only I had *that* kind of money, then people would finally shut up and listen when I talked.

Respect, I figured, was for sale. You just had to earn enough to buy it.

The whole thing started by accident, which, if you've been keeping score, is how most of my "big ideas" start. I was sitting in a Houston coffee shop one morning, nursing a burnt cup of something pretending to be espresso, when I met this guy. Older, tan, expensive watch, but wearing jeans.

We started talking. Turns out he was a real estate investor.

Now that rang a bell. I'd once tried to buy a ten-plex before grad school at Rice. Found it in the paper, back when people still used those and even put down earnest money. I was ready. I was going to be a mogul. Then my father, in all his booming Southern certainty, talked me out of it. Told me I was crazy, that I'd lose my shirt. So, I backed out. And I've been kicking myself ever since. So when this guy started talking about cap rates and cash flow, I was listening like he was Moses on the mountain. Then came the layoff. It's funny how the universe lines things up.

I'd been working at this investor relations firm, doing decent work, responsible, professional, all the words HR loves to see in an email. Then the economy took a nosedive, and suddenly, the company couldn't "afford" me. Translation: they couldn't afford anyone who wasn't indispensable, and apparently, that was not me.

It stung, especially since I had just bought a new BMW. The first one didn't count; it met its end courtesy of an eighteen-wheeler that didn't see me coming. Now, here I was again, jobless and car-rich.

No one likes to be fired. It's not just about the paycheck, though, trust me, watching the balance in your bank account nosedive is no small agony. It's something deeper. It's the slow, grinding realization that you weren't enough for somebody else's little world. You get the talk, the handshake, the fake sympathy, and then the walk of shame out the door with your dignity folded under your arm like a bad résumé.

For me, it wasn't the first time. Hell, it wasn't even the fifth. But this one, this one felt final. Something about it cracked through the last bit of my "I'll figure it out next time" optimism.
My ego, tender and inflated as a soap bubble, popped right there on the office floor.

On the drive home, I made a few decisions. That's what I do when the world knocks me down: I make decisions. Usually bad ones, but still decisions. I told myself, *I will never work for anyone else again.*

I will hold my damn tongue. I will play well in the sandbox. And most importantly, I will stop stepping into sandboxes that don't suit me in the first place.

When I finally got home, I sat on the sofa and stared at nothing. I thought about every office I'd been kicked out of, every boss I'd disappointed, and every time I'd promised myself this would be the last. There's a strange kind of peace that comes with hitting rock bottom so often, it starts to feel familiar, like an old roommate you can't quite get rid of.

That's when Roxy called. She liked the way I talked in meetings, my dark humor, my cynicism, my occasional bursts of brutal honesty. I think she found something oddly endearing about the train wreck that was me. We'd started talking more, mostly about writing. Turns out, she was a writer too.

Funny thing, so were a few of my other close friends. One was this old buddy from Houston who'd been writing poetry long before I even knew what vulnerability meant. The other was an American karate teacher I'd trained with years ago. A loudmouth, half-philosopher, half-warrior type who'd somehow seen something in me worth advancing to blue belt.

Roxy was different, though. She had this thing, this optimism that made me both admire her and want to roll my eyes. She'd listen to my rambling ideas, my half-baked theories about addiction, purpose, and pain, and instead of shooting them down, she'd say, "Why not write that?"

I'd laugh. "Because no one wants to hear the gospel according to a guy who just got fired again." But she'd push. She always pushed softly, persistently. So, we did it. We started writing. Talking. Dreaming. Scheming. It wasn't glamorous, two half-broken people trying to put words together like puzzle pieces, hoping it might mean something to someone someday. But something about it clicked. Her faith filled the gaps where my pessimism leaked through. And somewhere in that fragile beginning, the seed of our work, our *thing*, was planted.

I may not have had a job anymore, but I had something that felt like purpose. And that, I figured, was worth at least a few paychecks.

After a bit of time off, I decided to try my luck again. Perhaps, a route would pop out of nowhere. I decided to hit old friends, asking around.

"What do I do?" I asked my friend John one night, sitting in my half-empty apartment. John, who always seemed calmer than I deserved, shrugged. "You ever think of real estate? You'd be better off owning something instead of working for someone."

Owning. That word. It did something to me. So, I joined a local real estate club. Had no job, no experience, no savings, hell, less than zero net worth, but I showed up every Thursday with a notebook and the kind of enthusiasm only a desperate man can muster. Then, out of nowhere, came the call from my mom.

"Your grandmother's very ill," she said. "She wants to give each of the grandkids ten thousand. To avoid estate taxes."

Ten thousand dollars. To some people, that's nothing. To me, at that moment, it was the moon and stars. I'd blown gifts before, the last one partially funded the BMW that was now scrap metal, but this time, I swore it would be different.

So when the real estate club leader called and said, "Tad, I've got a deal for you, perfect fit," I didn't even blink. I met the seller, a wiry guy named Hank who smelled like cigarettes and roofing tar, and before long, I was signing papers.

$4,250 down.

$85,000 total.

And just like that, I was a landlord.

I can still remember the first time I pulled up to my new fourplex. Black 325i BMW, clean shirt, big grin, I thought I looked like a damn mogul. The tenants, however, were less impressed.

"Who's this guy?" I overheard one of them say. "Some rich white dude gonna screw us like the rest?"

Ah, the charm of first impressions.

Still, I dove in. Weekends were spent patching drywall, replacing sinks, fixing whatever the hell Sylvia, one of my more *vocal* tenants, had broken that week. She lived with her grandmother and brother in one of the downstairs units, and between the three of them, I think they kept the Houston plumbing industry alive.

I kept thinking to myself, *Maybe I'm not such a screw-up after all.*

During the week, I was back in the corporate grind. I'd managed to land another job, different title, same nonsense. My boss, Mario, liked to joke that I was "the terror of the office." He meant it as a compliment, I think. Or maybe not. Either way, I smiled and kept my mouth shut. Mostly.

The real estate thing gave me something my jobs never did: ownership, control, a weird sense of redemption. It was like taking all that frustration and finally hammering it into something solid. After a year, I refinanced the property, pulled out some cash, and bought a small house with a garage apartment. More tenants. More headaches. But more income, too.

Four years later, I sold the fourplex and used a 1031 exchange to buy two more homes in a rough-but-coming neighborhood. It wasn't glamorous, but it was progress. And when I finally sold one of those houses for $350,000, before taxes, of course, Uncle Sam always gets his cut, I just sat there staring at the check.

Ten thousand had turned into hundreds of thousands. Me. Tad Barnes. The guy who could barely keep a job. I thought about my grandmother that day. How that money was her last gift to us. How she never really believed I'd amount to much, and honestly, neither did I. But I did it. I built something. Maybe small, maybe scrappy, but *mine*.

I could almost hear her voice, soft but sharp as ever, "Don't get too proud now, Tad. Pride goeth before the fall." Yeah, Grandma. I know. But for once, could I maybe just enjoy standing a little taller before I trip again?

Because damn it, ten thousand dollars and a whole lot of stubbornness had built me a life.

And I was proud of that, even if I knew pride was a slippery rock.

******

It had been a long time since I'd thought about writing. Longer since I'd actually done it. The notebooks sat in a box somewhere, dog-eared pages, coffee stains, half-sentences that started brave and ended in defeat. I'd stopped pretending I was "on a break." The truth was, I'd quit. Writing had felt like another one of those things I couldn't sustain, like sobriety, jobs, and relationships. Everything that required consistency eventually demanded more than I had left to give.

Claire and I were walking that evening. One of our slow, aimless walks around the neighborhood, just enough to feel like movement, not enough to feel like exercise. The air was cool, the kind of crisp that wakes up your lungs and makes the world smell sharper. She was talking about something small, maybe a podcast or a book she'd read, when she said, "You used to write, right?" I don't know why that question hit so hard. Maybe because she said it like it was still true.

"Yeah," I said, kicking at a rock on the sidewalk. "Used to. That's the keyword."

She looked at me sideways, a quiet smile forming. "Used to? What happened?"

"Life," I said. "It happened. Got tired of my own words. Got tired of starting things I couldn't finish."

I shoved my hands in my jacket pockets. "There was a time when I thought writing would save me. Turns out, it just turned into another mirror showing me all the ways I was failing."

Claire didn't say anything right away. That was her thing, silence that didn't feel judgmental. She let you sit in your own words until you started to see what they were really saying.

After a while, she said softly, "You talk about it like it mattered. Like it still does."

I exhaled. "Maybe it does. Roxy, she's the one who got me into it seriously. We started this little writing and sharing thing together, back when I thought I could juggle things together. She believed in the whole dream of it. I believed in her belief. But then, you know, the usual, life picked me up, shook me around, and dropped me somewhere else. Writing just… slipped off the table."

Claire stopped walking and looked at me. The streetlight hit her face just enough to catch that calm, wry expression she gets when she's about to call me out gently. "So you stopped writing because life happened. But you're still living. So what's the excuse now?" That one stung because it was fair.

We started walking again, slower this time. The night hummed with that quiet sound only empty streets have. I could hear my own footsteps, my own breathing, my own resistance trying to talk me out of wanting anything again.

"You make it sound easy," I said.

"It's not," she replied. "But you already know what not doing it feels like. You could at least find out what doing it again feels like." Her words sank in somewhere deep. It wasn't a pep talk, more of a hand on the shoulder feeling, not a shove in the back.

That night, I couldn't sleep. I sat on the couch with my laptop open, the cursor blinking like it was mocking me. Claire had said she'd be my first reader if I ever wrote again. She even told me to send her whatever I came up with, no matter how bad, no matter how short.

"Just write," she said earlier that night, "and I'll hold you to it. Daily word counts, remember? You can hate me later." And God, I kind of did hate her for it because she was right.

So I started typing. Not much. Just a paragraph. A shaky start about a man sitting alone, afraid to open his own life back up.

It felt clumsy. Awkward. I won't lie, something did happen. I felt my brain shift gears, like an old engine trying to turn over. I felt that faint, familiar heat in my chest, the one that says, *This still matters.* I didn't tell her right away. But the next night, when she called, I admitted I'd written something.

Her voice lit up, calm but sure. "Good," she said. "Tomorrow, do it again." And somehow, that small act, her listening, her quiet belief, brought something back to life in me I thought was long gone.

Long walks and late-night talks had done what self-help books and therapists couldn't. They'd awakened the part of me that still wanted to create, to tell the truth in my own words, even if those words sometimes scared the hell out of me. Maybe that was what a chunk of trying to heal looked like. Not fireworks or grand revelations. Just two people walking under a quiet sky, talking about forgotten dreams, and daring them to breathe again.

Chapter Seventeen

I always dreaded this. Not because of the coffin-sized space, or the weird beeps, clanks, and chirps that sound similar to some alien machinery tuning up. Not even because of the cost, thank you, insurance, for once. No. What I dreaded was the possibility of falling asleep mid-scan, snoring into the microphone, and having the technician gently chastise me over the intercom. "Sir, please stay still." It happened once, years ago. My humiliation lasted longer than the scan.

Today was MRI day again. Lucky me. The ritual was all too familiar, the same battery of questions, the same clipboard shoved across the counter, the same "name, date of birth, address" song-and-dance. My name, "Tankard Rankin Jaehrling," stretched across the paper. Way too long. I gave up signing that monstrosity years ago and settled on a squiggle. It started in grad school when I realized I didn't have time for all those letters. Now it was part of the brand: "Tankard" the man, "squiggle" the signature.

They called my name. "Mr. Jaehrling?" God, I hated that. That was my father's name. "Tad," I corrected automatically.

The waiting room was a cold shade of beige. Medical offices always have that same tired palette, like they're trying not to offend anyone's sensibilities. I sat there nursing a large coffee that had already gone lukewarm, waiting for the inevitable. My impatience gnawed at me. I hated waiting. I had too much to do; emails, errands, and some half-finished plumbing work at the new house I'd just bought in Dallas. The house had character, by which I mean it had a thousand small repairs.

I pulled out my phone and called the repairman. "Hola, Claudio. ¿Cómo estás?" We exchanged pleasantries. My Spanish wasn't perfect, but I was proud of it.

"Ok, no quiero pagar más que doscientos dólares, ¿ok?" I told him. I could almost hear him smiling through the phone.

When I hung up, the woman next to me, maybe mid-fifties, looked impressed. "Wow," she said. "You did that amazingly well. I studied for two years, and I couldn't do what you just did."

I shrugged. "I've got a musical ear. Helps with languages."

We chatted for a bit, the basics, weekend plans, the world's current state of chaos, the weather (because there's always the weather). I liked talking to strangers. You could reveal small slivers of yourself and then walk away without consequence. Finally, the receptionist perked up. "The technician will be right out."

And then she appeared, Paris. That was her name. She was striking, with long black dreadlocks and a quiet confidence that filled the room. "Hi, I'm Paris," she said, extending her hand.

"Tad," I replied, grateful she didn't go for the "Mr. Jaehrling" nonsense.

"Come on back, and we'll get you started."

The MRI room was sterile and green, humming with low mechanical life. The machine sat there in the center like some giant, hungry donut waiting to swallow me whole. A bench stood against the right wall, and four folded gowns rested neatly on a table to the left.

"Does it matter which way I put this on?" I asked, holding one up. "And, uh, underwear?"

181

Paris smiled. "You're fine, hon."

She went over the instructions. Don't move, stay still, breathe evenly. Then she asked what kind of music I wanted. "Top 40," I said.

She raised an eyebrow. "You sure? It helps if you're calm."

"Alright," I sighed. "Classical it is." She moved with that quiet precision that people in healthcare seem to master.

"I like your style," I said as she adjusted the straps.

"Thank you, Tad. I like yours too." The compliment hit me harder than expected, maybe because she said my name. Maybe because I hadn't heard warmth in someone's voice like that all day. And then, it was show time. They slid me into the machine, headfirst. The plastic bracket came down over my skull like some medieval restraint.

"Do I have to wear this thing?" I asked.

"It's part of the drill."

I groaned. "Figures." The machine roared to life. Burps, chirps, clicks, taps, wheezes, whistles, each sound added a pinch of anxiety in my gut. The classical music bled faintly through the noise. Bach, maybe. Or Beethoven. I couldn't tell. The notes tried their best to make this feel civilized, but there's nothing civilized about lying flat in a tube, unable to scratch an itch near your left eye.

I stared ahead at the bland, white interior. Nothing to see. Nowhere to look. Just my thoughts and the sound of industry. And that's when the mind began to wander, because where else could it go? I thought about the disease. My old enemy. Multiple freaking sclerosis. MS. It had stormed into my life like a thief, stealing without warning. One morning, I woke up and couldn't see out of my left eye. Two days later, the vision came back, sort of. Fuzzy, compromised, like a TV with bad reception.

MS, you bitch, I thought. You took my goddamn life.

But then another voice inside me asked, *Or did it give you one?* I swallowed hard. That thought lingered for a while.

The thing about lying still in that damn MRI capsule is, it gives you time to think. Too much time, really. The kind that corners you in your own head and starts unspooling everything you've been avoiding. Somewhere between the third and fourth round of beeps, I started thinking about my old life. If you could call it that.

Cocktail-laden nights, house parties with more booze than oxygen. Meaningless, trippy flings that blurred one into another, people whose names I couldn't remember, whose faces I sometimes still saw in dreams I didn't want. Conversations that went nowhere but still haunted me anyway. Was that really a life? Or just a long, slow suicide disguised as fun?

It all changed after the diagnosis. Those two words, multiple sclerosis, dropped like a grenade in the middle of my little circus. The doctors, the referrals, the "state agency assistance," the suggestion to check out AA. "It might help," they'd said, as if sobriety could fix brain lesions.

And yet... here I was.

A tear slid down my cheek before I even realized it. One of those rogue tears that sneaks up when you're trying too hard to be composed. After this was over, I wanted to tell Paris how I felt. I didn't *have* to. There was no moral obligation. No therapist's nudge. But I *wanted* to. She seemed like someone

183

who'd actually listen. No judgment, no awkward silences. Just human-to-human understanding. There was something about her calm steadiness that disarmed me completely. Maybe I just needed someone to see me as something other than "the patient."

Somewhere between the burps and clanks of the machine, my thoughts drifted again, because that's what they always did. My mind's a pinball machine; it never stops bouncing. Would I write about this? Probably. Everything became material sooner or later.

And then, Brianna.

God, Brianna.

August 1998. I was thirty, and she was eighteen. She was sitting in that diner with her blonde friend, legs draped across the bench like she owned the world, half-seduced by her own youth. I was hooked immediately. Wasn't that how "true love" worked? You see someone, and bam, you just *know*?

Oh, how I liked that girl. Maybe even loved her, though what did I know about love back then? I was drunk half the time and emotionally stunted the other half. Back then, I thought love was a combination of adrenaline, alcohol, and good lighting. I cried over Brianna more nights than I care to admit, sitting in my crappy apartment, chain-smoking and listening to love songs written for people who could actually sustain relationships. I was convinced she didn't care. Turns out, she did.

She'd hinted at a few casual encounters, three, to be exact, but I'd said no. Why? Because I wanted to "do it right." I wanted dinner first. The wine. The illusion of romance. I wanted to pretend I was capable of something normal. Nothing came of it.

Now she's in Los Angeles, happy, engaged, living some filtered, sunlit life. I've seen the pictures.

I tell myself I'm happy for her, but mostly, I just feel old. Ah, Brianna, the tragedy of the unlived tragedy. The machine buzzed louder, and I let out a soft laugh that no one could hear. This was absurd. My whole life had been a mix of absurdities stitched together by bad timing.

The thoughts came faster now: my book, my body, my hair, my so-called future. Random flashes of ambition and loss colliding in a small, white capsule that sounded like a construction site. How many hours had I been in here? It felt like ten. In reality, three. Three long, grinding hours of mechanical percussion and classical music, trying to calm my nerves.

When they finally pulled me out, I felt like a half-baked loaf of bread, a bit pale, sweaty, done. I changed quickly, met Paris in the hallway. She had that same patient smile.

"Paris, I'm going to put you in my book," I blurted.

She raised an eyebrow. "Absolutely."

"What should I call you?"

"I think you know the drill," she said, smirking.

I grinned. "You got it. And hey, give my info to your brother in L.A., yeah? The literary agent?"

"I will, Tad," she said, pulling her mask down. It startled me a bit, seeing someone's whole face was a rarity in those pandemic days. She had kind eyes.

"How cool," I said. "I can actually see your face now." And just like that, I felt strangely triumphant. Another MRI done.

Another disc of my brain's weird geography in hand. Another reminder that I was still alive.

The weekend was quiet. I cleaned the house. I hate cleaning. Always have. But I hate spending money even more, and the idea of hiring someone to do it felt extravagant. So, I did it myself. Made sense, right? Afterward, I crashed on the couch, stared at the ceiling for a while, then dragged myself to an AA meeting.

Monday rolled around, bland and unremarkable. The kind of day that's so normal it almost feels comforting. Mondays have that way of offering a reset button after the chaos of a weekend. By mid-morning, I was knee-deep in spreadsheets, trying to convince myself I was productive. Then I stretched, picked up my phone, and noticed the missed calls.

Three of them. All from the MS clinic. Great. Never a good sign when a medical office calls more than once. One voicemail. "Please call us as soon as possible."

"Mr. Jaehrling," the nurse began. "The MRI found some more lesions." My stomach dropped. Lesions. That word again. The invisible fingerprints of a disease that wouldn't quit.

"We found lesions," she continued, "and the doctor's prescribing a two-week steroid regimen. We've called it into your pharmacy." No empathy, no soft cushioning. Just another announcement that my body was quietly betraying me. Hot damn. MS strikes again.

Couldn't I just have a *normal* life? One stretch of time where nothing went wrong? But no, my track record said otherwise. I'd been born unlucky, apparently. As a kid, I was the poster child for ailments, asthma, hay fever, pneumonia that almost took me out. My mom, Kitty, still tells that story like a trauma badge. "You almost died," she'd say, her voice still shaky decades later.

Then came the thick glasses, the 'cokers,' as the other kids called them. Coke-bottle lenses that made me look like a bug-eyed alien. And kids are cruel. They don't need reasons to mock, but boy, they loved that one.

High school got marginally better once the bullies aged out or flunked out. Then college came, and the cycle reset, new faces, same mockery. Did it ever end?

There was a small reprieve during business school. God, I loved that phase. My people. My tribe of pseudo-intellectuals pontificating about global markets while downing cheap beer on Thursday nights. We solved the world's problems before collapsing into plates of greasy Mexican food. Those were good days. After B-school, I ran off to California chasing the Hollywood mirage. Why not? I was good-looking enough, smart enough, charming enough. I could act.

I was also $40,000 in debt and allergic to poverty. That's a bad combo in L.A. I came close once, my "big break," a commercial that actually won a gold Clio. And then I chickened out. Went into management instead. My second-favorite path, a safer one, indeed. And since I was living in California, I figured I'd do what Californians do: reinvent myself.

LASIK surgery? Check. They said I was too young for it. I did it anyway. Next came the fitness kick. I was going to get into the best shape of my life, find the hottest bride I could, and finally have it all. And for a while, it worked. No six-pack, but enough definition to turn heads. Good teeth, good hair, a decent face, until that bald spot started mocking me in the mirror.

So I fixed that too. Hair transplant. Cost me a fortune, didn't even cover the whole damn thing. Still a patch left. I obsessed over it anyway. Perfection was always just out of reach. And now, sitting there with a new lesion in my brain and an old scar on my scalp, I couldn't help but laugh.

Why couldn't I get any breaks?

Chapter Eighteen

Before Al left us, I remember life pulled the rug from beneath our feet by gifting us the pandemic, and with it came more misery. It started with the damn alert on the radio. "Harris County has been upgraded to Code One, Red." Just like that, it was official: the world had shut down.

One month before, I'd finally landed a job that didn't make me feel like I was being auctioned off to the highest bidder. No sales, no quotas, no fake smiles while someone told me why they couldn't "move forward right now." This gig wasn't glamorous, but it was steady. There was quiet. I could breathe without pretending to be excited about another spreadsheet. And then, the world decided to collapse.

I was halfway into my work clothes that morning, coffee half-drunk, tie crooked, when the alert hit the airwaves. I just stood there, mug in hand, staring at the TV like it had personally betrayed me.

"Only essential workers permitted to leave home." Well, I sure as hell wasn't essential. Not in any category that mattered.

Rage simmered somewhere under my ribs, that old familiar kind that had nowhere to go but inward. I grabbed my keys anyway, stormed out, and got in the car. I wasn't even sure where I was going, maybe nowhere. Maybe everywhere.

The stereo went up, *full blast*. Music so loud it drowned out the world. I tore down I-45 like an Indy 500 wannabe, weaving through lanes like I was chasing something invisible. Cars honked, brakes squealed, it just didn't matter. I had shit to do, even if I didn't know what it was. Then, of course, the universe decided to check me. One idiot driver cut across the lane too slowly, and I didn't have time to stop.

Crunch.

"Oh, shit."

We pulled over, her face already a storm cloud of irritation. She was polite but tight-lipped. We exchanged info, called the cops, and went through the whole miserable routine. When the officer showed up, he sighed like a man who'd already had a hundred of these today.

"I'm not giving you a ticket," he said flatly. "Got too much going on right now." I nodded. The woman didn't look pleased. Couldn't blame her.

I drove off, knuckles white on the wheel. Somewhere between guilt and relief, I laughed out loud, one of those short, bitter laughs that die in your throat. "Just perfect, Tad," I muttered. "Real smooth start to the apocalypse."

The days that followed blurred together.

Work from home, eat, stare at walls, wonder if this was it. Life reduced to waiting.

The silence was the worst part. You could only pretend things were fine for so long before you heard the truth echoing back at you.

My mom, of course, was still pretending everything was wonderful. She was losing her memory, her logic, her ability to connect dots, but she held on to optimism like a religion. Positive. Sure. Right up until it kills you.

I came from a family of professional self-deceivers. My dad could build an entire reality around denial, and my mom? She believed every fairy tale that promised a happy ending as long as she didn't have to face what came before it.

When her fairy tales fell apart, she drank. When they somehow held together, she still drank. And me? I pretended I was different. But there it was, the same blood, same habits, same fears dressed up as control.

The call came one morning. I was at my desk, writing down the day's "plan." (A joke, really. I was organizing ways to avoid work.) My phone rang. Emma.

My stomach dropped. Calls from Emma were never good.

"Hey, Tad, I need your help," she said, breathless. "Your mom's not doing well. She can't hold down food. I tried Pedialyte, but she spits it up. I wanted to take her to the doctor, but they said she might have COVID, and they don't want to take a chance." Of course they didn't. No one wanted to take a chance.

"Alright," I said, trying to keep my voice steady. "I'll take care of it." I walked outside before the panic could corner me. My hands were shaking. I dialed the doctor's office. Rings. More rings. Then that robotic voice, *"Press one for scheduling, press two for billing…"*

"Dr. Robinson's office," a woman finally answered.

"Yes, this is Tad Jaehrling. I need to speak to someone about my mom, Kitty Jaehrling."

"Kitty Jaer…?"

"Jaehrling," I said, grinding my teeth. "J-A-E-H-R-L-I-N-G."

"Okay. Date of birth?"

"November fifteenth, nineteen-forty."

191

Click-click on a keyboard. "And your relationship to the patient?"

"She's my mom. I have medical power of attorney."

(One of those life titles you never want but end up getting anyway.)

"What can we do for you?"

"She can't hold down food," I said. "Been throwing up non-stop. We need to see the doctor today."

"Hold, please." The line went silent, replaced by that god-awful New Age hold music. Flutes and water sounds. I stood there in my driveway, listening to what sounded similar to a spa commercial for people losing their minds. Finally, she came back. "Mr. Jaehrling, it says your mother came in, but the doctor couldn't see her because of COVID."

"What?"

"Yes, the doctor can't see her until we get the test results."

"But she hasn't had a test yet," I snapped. "And it takes three to five days to get results! What good will that be if she's dead by then?"

"I'm sorry, sir, that's the policy."

My pulse throbbed in my temples. Claire was standing near the sofa. She had come for a visit. She was watching me with that expression she wore whenever she saw I was about to self-combust, like she was quietly timing the countdown before I blew.

"Look," I said, pacing now. "Chantelle, can I call you Chantelle?"

"That's fine, sir."

192

"Listen, my mom doesn't have COVID. She hasn't seen anyone except my dad, the caregiver, and me. None of us has symptoms."

"I'm sorry, Mr. Jaehrling," she repeated, the script in her voice as dry as an instruction manual. "But that's the best we can do."

And that's when I snapped. It wasn't even gradual. One second, I was talking like a reasonable adult, and the next I was roaring into the phone like a man who'd finally had enough of bureaucracy, fear, and goddamned policies that put procedure over people.

"Let me tell you something," I said, my voice trembling but steady in its fury. "If my mom dies because your office wouldn't see her, because you were too damn scared of a maybe… You can rest assured I'll sue the goddamned shit out of you. And don't think I'm bluffing. I'm crazy as hell, and I could use the money!"

Silence. Even the birds in the trees seemed to stop chirping. I could feel Claire's eyes on me, not judging, not interrupting, just there.

Then, the woman's voice, soft as tissue, said, "Could you hold, please?"

The flutes came back. God help me, I wanted to drive over there and smash the speaker playing that music. I looked at Claire, who was leaning against the wall now, hands tucked into the pockets of her cardigan.

After a few minutes, the line clicked again. "Mr. Jaehrling," Chantelle said, her tone different now, careful, conciliatory. "We do have a relationship with John Wesley Hospital. Could you take her there today?"

"Now we're talking," I said, exhaling like a man who'd just won a small, ugly war. I ended the call and just stood there, adrenaline still burning in my veins. My hands were shaking, and for a moment, I didn't trust my own voice.

Claire came closer, resting a gentle hand on my arm. "You did good," she said quietly. "You fought for her." I stared at her, this calm, infuriatingly centered woman who somehow managed to make chaos feel less like a hurricane and more like a wind you could walk through.

"Yeah, well," I muttered, trying to play it off. "I'm just getting started."

She gave me a smile that never failed to disarm me. Then she took out her phone, already dialing. "Let me talk to them," she said. "You've done the heavy lifting. I'll handle the logistics."

And she did. Calmly, professionally, without a hint of anger or panic. She spoke with the hospital staff in that clear, composed tone of hers, the way I never could. By the time she was done, my mom had an appointment, a bed reserved, and a note on her chart that said "urgent."

I just stood there, watching her. That's the thing about Claire. She doesn't need to shout to be powerful. She doesn't need to threaten lawsuits or use sarcasm as a shield. She just handles it.

I realized something I hadn't wanted to admit out loud: I needed someone like her in my life. Not because she fixed things. But because, when the world went sideways, she reminded me that maybe, it could still be put back together.

That evening, Al, Emma, my mom, and I drove to John Wesley Hospital. The place was chaos; everyone in masks, nurses darting around like ghosts behind plexiglass. They took my mom's vitals, did the test, told us to wait.

Two days later, the results came in.

Negative. Just like I'd said.

I called the doctor's office, half wanting to gloat, half just exhausted.

"She's fine," I said. "Thanks for nothing." Then I hung up and sat in silence for a long while, letting the relief crawl through me.

The world was falling apart. Jobs were disappearing, people were dying, and everyone was scared. But for once, something had gone right. Mom was okay. And for that one moment, I could breathe again.

Chapter Nineteen

I wasn't expecting her to actually come over. We'd joked about it for weeks, "One day I'll stop by and see the famous writer's den," she'd said. I laughed it off. Didn't correct her on the *writer* part, even though I'd given that up months ago. But that Saturday, just after lunch, there she was.

I heard the knock before I even had time to hide the evidence, the half-eaten pizza box, the stack of unopened mail, the coffee mug that looked like it had hosted a science experiment. When I opened the door, Claire was standing there with a bunch of flowers in one hand and a plastic container in the other. Her hair was pulled back, her sweatshirt loose, her eyes bright as if she'd been laughing at her own private joke.

"I come bearing gifts," she said, lifting the container. "Cupcakes. Homemade. Don't get excited. They're ugly, but they taste good."

"Story of my life," I said. She smiled and handed them over, then stepped inside. And immediately, I saw it, the tiny flicker in her eyes as she looked around, the hesitation. I'd seen it before. The polite scan people do when they realize you live alone, and it *shows*. The curtains half-pinned, the couch that had seen better decades, the smell of something like dust and regret.

I could feel myself starting to fill the silence. "Yeah, it's not exactly *Better Homes & Gardens*. I was going for more of a 'post-divorce chic meets existential crisis' vibe." Claire didn't laugh right away, which made it worse. I shoved my hands into my pockets, ready for the usual pity smile.

But instead, she said softly, "I like this color."

"What?" She was staring at the wall by the window, the one I'd painted a dull blue years ago because it was on sale and the label said *Pacific Dusk*. I'd hated it ever since. Too cold for my eyes.

"This blue," she said. "It's kind of beautiful. It looks like the sky right before it rains. The kind of color that holds its breath." I blinked. No one had ever said that before. Most people didn't even notice the wall, or if they did, they said it made the room feel small.

"You're serious?" I said.

She nodded, still studying it. "Yeah. It's moody. I like moody. Feels like someone actually *lives* here."

I let out a laugh, partly out of relief. "You mean someone *survives* here."

"Same thing sometimes," she said, shrugging, and walked over to place the flowers on the table. I watched her move through the room, like she wasn't seeing the mess at all. Just the life in it. The photo of my parents on the shelf, the half-written notes on the counter, the cheap candle I'd been burning down to nothing.

"Damn," I said finally, shaking my head. "You're dangerous."

She looked back. "How so?"

"You walk into a man's mess and make him believe it's art." That earned me the quiet, knowing laugh, the one that always came from the back of her throat. "I just see things as they are," she said. "Not how they're supposed to be."

We sat down after that. She poured coffee, I opened the cupcakes, and for a while, the silence between us wasn't awkward; it was easy to breathe in. Like we'd agreed to stop pretending for a minute. She took a bite and said, "You know, these could use more sugar."

I smirked. "Finally, something I can fix."

She grinned, wiping her hands. "Don't. They're perfect like this. Not everything has to be sweet." Something in that line hit deeper than it should have. I didn't say anything. Just looked at the blue wall again, with that stormy, waiting color, and thought maybe for once, she was right.

Chapter Twenty

It wasn't supposed to be one of those days. I was just running errands: milk, cat food, and some goddamn paper towels that never seemed to last. Nothing epic. Just me, my old beat-up bike, and the low hum of Houston traffic under a syrupy sunset.

I shouldn't have taken the bike. I knew that. The front brake had been whining for weeks, and I kept saying I'd fix it "tomorrow," which, like most of my tomorrows, never came. But I needed the air, the motion, something to shake loose the static that had been buzzing in my head all week.

Claire's voice was still there, tucked somewhere in that noise. "Maybe you should try being still for once, Tad." Stillness. Right. I'd tried that once; it was called depression. So I rode. The wind cut against my face, humid and heavy, sticking to my skin. I remember thinking, *this feels like swimming through soup.*

My head wasn't on the road. It was back with her, the way she looked that morning, laughing at my ridiculous attempt to make coffee while half-asleep. The way she tucked a loose strand of hair behind her ear, slow, absentminded. How I wanted to reach over and do it for her. That thought lingered a little too long. Long enough that I didn't notice the white delivery van nosing out of the alleyway until it was too damn late.

I swerved hard left, instinct, not thought. The front tire clipped the curb. There was a loud pop. Was it my tire or my bone, maybe both? Suddenly, I was airborne. Then came the sound. Metal scraping pavement. My head hitting something that wasn't soft. A brief, searing pain up my left side, and then silence took a bow.

The world flipped. The orange sky traded places with the asphalt. My body skidded, the smell of burned rubber and blood mixing into something acrid and metallic. I lay there, flat on my back, staring up at a palm tree that looked almost peaceful against the fading sky. And the first thing that hit me wasn't fear, wasn't pain.

It was *her.*

Not my mom, not my father, not God… *Claire.*

I don't even remember reaching for my phone, but there it was in my hand, the screen cracked, her name glowing through the spiderweb of fractures. I hit call. My fingers were shaking so hard I almost dropped it.

"Hey, you okay?" she answered. Her voice, steady as ever, threaded through the chaos.

"I…" I couldn't catch my breath. Everything inside me was rattling. "Claire…"

"Tad? What's wrong? Where are you?"

"Bike," I muttered. "Crash… think I'm…"

"Tad! Jesus, are you hurt? Stay with me, okay? Tell me where you are!" But her voice was slipping. Everything around me was dimming, as if someone was slowly turning down the volume on life itself. My eyes were open, but the world was fading.

Then, all went black.

When I woke up, I was sure I'd died and landed somewhere between a hospital and a hell designed by interior decorators

200

who hated color. Everything was white. A monitor was beeping steadily near my head, and the air smelled like antiseptic and lemon cleaner. My mouth carried the taste of dust and some fated regret.

Then I saw her, sitting beside me in a plastic chair, her head bent, hair spilling over her face. She was holding a cup of coffee that had probably gone cold hours ago. Her sneakers were untied. There was a small crease between her brows, even in sleep. For a long time, I didn't move. I just watched her.

This woman, this calm, maddeningly grounded woman, had somehow found her way into my orbit and refused to leave. And now she was sitting there, in a hospital room that smelled of bleach and bad food, because of me. I shifted, and pain shot through my shoulder, my ribs, my everything. The monitor blipped faster. She stirred immediately.

"Tad?" Her voice cracked a little. "Oh, thank God." She leaned forward, eyes wide, scanning me like she expected to find missing pieces. "You scared the hell out of me."

I tried to smile. "Yeah, well... figured I'd test the hospital system. See if it still works."

She exhaled, half-laugh, half-sob. "Don't joke about that."

"Sorry," I croaked. My throat felt strangely sandy. "Did they, uh... did they fix the bike?"

She blinked, incredulous. "The bike? Tad, you nearly cracked your skull open."

"Guess I needed to clear my head," I said, voice rasping. Claire just shook her head, biting back a smile she didn't want me to see.

I reached out weakly, motioning her closer. "Claire..."

"What is it? Do you need water? Should I get the nurse?"

"No." My hand hovered midair until she caught it. "Just… sit. Close."

Her expression softened immediately. "Okay." She pulled the chair closer until her knees brushed the side of the bed. Her hand was warm, which felt good. I looked at her and felt something unclench inside me.

"Knew you'd come," I murmured.

She squeezed my hand. "Of course I came. You scared me half to death, you idiot."

I laughed or tried to. It came out as a wheeze. "Guess I still got that effect on women."

She rolled her eyes but didn't let go. "You're impossible."

"Yeah," I said softly. "But you're still here." Her thumb moved slowly across the back of my hand. I felt she understood me. Why did it matter, though? Why did it matter if I mattered to her?

Was I falling for her? I mean, why would she fall for me… I am no short of a mess. She perhaps pities me; that is why she is here. She feels sorry for me.

"Tad, I am glad nothing happened to you…" Her eyes were glistening.

"Would you mind if something happened to me?"

"I don't know how I would have dealt with it… My world trembled when I heard your voice… I…" She paused to catch her breath. "I am happy you are in one piece…" She smiled. I felt her grip tighten around my hand.

"Yeah, me too."

They released me two days later. Bruised ribs, mild concussion, some spectacular road rash, and a newfound appreciation for gravity. The doctor said I was lucky. I told him luck had nothing to do with it; I had Claire. She'd been there through every minute, hovering, fussing, steady as a heartbeat. I hadn't asked her to. She just did. That's how she was.

When we got back to my place, I tried to wave her off. "You don't have to stay, Claire. I'm fine. Really."

She gave me that raised eyebrow, arms-crossed look that could stop a train. "You can barely stand up without swearing, Tad. You're not fine."

"Well, swearing is part of my recovery plan."

"I'll make you some tea," she said, completely ignoring me.

I watched her move around my kitchen. She found the old kettle, somehow knew which drawer held the tea bags. "You really need better lighting in here," she said.

"I was going for 'mysterious bachelor who reads by candlelight,'" I muttered.

She turned, smiling faintly. "You nailed 'bachelor.' Still working on the mysterious part."

I laughed, then winced. "Ow. Don't make me laugh. Hurts to breathe."

"Sorry," she said, not sounding sorry at all. "You're just... accident-prone but worth it."

"Worth it, huh?" I leaned back on the couch, feigning smugness but secretly filing those words away somewhere sacred. She brought me tea and a small plate of the cupcakes she'd made earlier in the week, the same ones she'd brought the first time she came over. She set them down beside me, then crouched to my level.

"You need to take your meds," she said softly.

"Yes, Nurse Claire."

"Don't start." She opened the bottle and handed me two pills with that kind of gentle firmness you don't argue with. Her fingers brushed mine. I pretended not to notice, but my pulse had other plans. Afterward, she helped me adjust the pillows, tucking the blanket around me as if I was something fragile. Nobody had done that for me in, I couldn't even remember.

"You really don't have to do this," I said again.

"Do what?"

"Play Florence Nightingale."

"I'm not playing anything, Tad." She smiled, but her eyes stayed serious. "You scared me. You don't get to brush that off." The words hit harder than I expected. Nobody ever admitted being scared for me. Most people just assumed I'd land on my feet until I didn't.

So, I did the only thing I knew how to do: make a joke. "Scared, huh? You sure it's not just my irresistible charm?"

She smirked. "Definitely the concussion talking." But when she looked away, I caught it, the flicker of something softer beneath the sarcasm. We spent the evening half-watching old movies. She sat close enough that I could feel the warmth of her arm against mine. Every now and then, she'd glance over to make sure I was still awake, still breathing, still *there*.

At some point, I must've dozed off. I woke to the sound of her voice, talking to someone on the phone, her sister, maybe. The light was dim, the room hazy with quiet. "He's resting," she was saying. "No, he's okay. Just bruised up. Yeah… I'll stay here tonight. He shouldn't be alone."

I didn't move. I didn't want to break the moment. She hung up, then turned toward me. "You awake?"

"Maybe," I said, voice rough. "You really staying?"

"Yeah," she said simply. "You'd just try to get up in the middle of the night and break something else."

"Fair point."

She smiled faintly, then moved the blanket up over my chest. "Go back to sleep, Tad." Her hand lingered on my arm for just a beat too long, not romantic, but something was changing. There was a tenderness there that neither of us could quite name yet.

I lay there, half-conscious, listening to her breathing beside me, and it hit me, I didn't want her to leave. Not tomorrow, not the next day. Maybe not ever, but will I say this out loud, probably not. At least not today.

Somewhere between the pain and the pills, I drifted again. The last thing I remember before sleep took me was her humming softly under her breath, a tune I didn't recognize, but one that made the room feel less empty.

When I woke in the morning, sunlight was spilling through the blinds, and there she was, curled in the armchair, dozing lightly, hair mussed, still in yesterday's jeans. And it struck me, with absolute clarity, I was falling for her.

Not in the way you fall when you're drunk or lonely, but the slow, unguarded way, the kind that sneaks up on you until you realize you're already in too deep.

Shit…

Chapter Twenty One

Claire and I decided to go down to Houston for a few weeks to help Emma out because she was having a hard time managing Mom by herself.

The house feels different now, like somebody opened a window that had been sealed shut for years, and the air finally remembered how to move. Claire and Emma started splitting the care shifts for Kitty a few weeks ago, and somehow, without planning it, a rhythm settled in.

Claire comes in the mornings, bright and unhurried, moving through the house as if she's known it forever. She hums when she makes breakfast, reads out snippets of the news, and talks to Kitty like she's right there listening. Then Emma arrives in the afternoons, practical, warm, a little bossy in the way older sisters tend to be. She and Claire tag-team the transitions like it's choreography. I mostly stay out of the way, which I've learned is sometimes the best kind of help.

Evenings are my favorite, though. By then, Kitty's usually drowsy, her small body tucked under that faded quilt she loves. Claire makes tea; Emma flips through the channels until she lands on some old Western, *Gunsmoke*, *Bonanza*, one of those. The kind of shows Dad used to watch when the world was simpler, or maybe just smaller.

And I sit there, somewhere between observer and participant, pretending to focus on the screen while my brain quietly tries to figure out what the hell is happening to me.

The first night it hit me was during *High Noon*. Claire was sitting on the edge of the couch, her legs tucked under her, her attention half on the movie, half on Kitty breathing in the next room. Emma had just made popcorn, the real kind, on the stove, and the smell of butter filled the whole place. It was domestic. The kind of normal I never thought I'd want, let alone get to live in.

And the thing that got me wasn't the movie or the popcorn. It was the quiet. Not the awkward, suffocating kind I used to drown in. This was the other kind, the steady, living quiet of people who didn't need to fill every space with noise to prove they belonged. I caught myself watching Claire. The way she smiled faintly at the screen, the way she nudged Emma when the sheriff did something noble and stupid.

I didn't say anything, but something inside me cracked open a little.

When the movie ended, the credits rolling over that slow western score, Claire turned to me.

"You like those old cowboy films?"

"Not really," I said. "They're predictable. Guy does something dumb in the name of honor, gets shot, and everyone calls him a hero."

She smirked. "You sound like you've thought about this a lot."

"I had a dad who thought John Wayne was a philosopher."

Emma laughed softly from the recliner. "He kind of was."

"Sure," I said. "If your philosophy involves dying alone on principle."

Claire shook her head, still smiling. "Or standing your ground when everyone else runs." I looked at her for a moment, the steady calm in her eyes, the kind of conviction that didn't need a spotlight. "You'd last about five minutes in an old Western," I said.

She shrugged. "Maybe. But I'd still show up."

That stuck with me, *I'd still show up.* It's the kind of thing that sounds simple until you realize how few people actually do it. When Emma left that night, the house dimmed down to that late-hour stillness. Claire stayed behind a little longer, helping me clean up. She washed the mugs, and I dried them. We didn't talk much. We didn't have to.

At one point, she reached for a towel and brushed my arm. Just a second of contact, but my chest tightened like a pulled stitch. "Thanks for letting us take over your space," she said quietly.

I shook my head. "You didn't take over. You just... made it make sense again."

She looked at me then, not searching, not trying to fix me, just *seeing* me. That unnerved me more than I wanted to admit. She smiled lightly. "You're getting better at this, you know."

"At what?"

"Letting people in."

I scoffed. "Don't get ahead of yourself. I'm just tolerating you because you bring cupcakes."

She laughed. "Sure, Tad. Whatever you say." When she left, I stood in the doorway and watched her walk to her car. The air was cold, the sky that kind of bruised blue that comes right before midnight.

Inside, the TV flickered in the empty living room, Kitty's soft breathing steady down the hall. And for the first time in a long time, the silence didn't feel like punishment.

It felt like peace, and tomorrow, we'd go back to Dallas, knowing we'd be back again soon. And we were.

Chapter Twenty Two

It was a long drive from Dallas to Houston. Three and a half hours on a good day, maybe five if I stopped at Buc-ee's, which I always did, because, well, who can resist a beaver promising world-class bathrooms and brisket sandwiches? The problem was, there was no place to sit in those damn stores. You can buy a fire pit, a onesie, and a fifty-pound bag of deer corn, but you can't sit your ass down for five minutes. A one-man crusade, that. I'd die on that hill.

But that day, it wasn't about pit stops. It was about time, how fast it was running, and how much I wanted to slow it down. I'd built something resembling a life in Dallas. Somehow managed to shake off the ghosts of Houston; the coke-bottle glasses, the kids who made sport of my existence, the long shadow of inferiority that trailed me well into adulthood. Dallas had become home. My reinvention project. Now, heading back south felt like walking straight into the lion's den after you'd already escaped.

Claire came with me. I didn't ask her to. She just said, "You shouldn't do this alone," and threw her overnight bag in the backseat like it was the most natural thing in the world. And it was, at least, by then, it was.

We didn't talk much on the drive. We didn't have to. She rested her hand on my arm sometimes, thumb tracing small circles near my wrist. Every so often, she'd reach for the coffee between us, take a sip, and pass it back. That small rhythm, her touch, her silence was the only thing keeping me from unraveling completely.

When the skyline of Houston came into view, that oily gleam of humidity and concrete, I felt my chest tighten. I tried to joke. "Welcome to my personal hell," I said.

Claire just squeezed my hand. "We'll get through it," she said.

The traffic near the Medical Center was its usual nightmare; horns blaring, ambulances cutting through lanes. Houston drivers were born impatient and raised reckless. Dallas drivers were better; they'd told me so themselves, usually by honking at me when I didn't move fast enough. We finally made it to John Wesley Hospital. I rolled down my window at the valet stand, only for the guy to wave us off. Of course. So I found a spot two blocks away and parked myself.

By the time we got inside, the front desk felt like airport security. Who are you here to see? For how long? What's the check-in time? What's the checkout time? Mask, gloves, gown. I wanted to ask if they needed a DNA sample, too. They told me Mom had been moved to hospice. I felt something inside me crack. Hospice. The word no one wants to hear but everyone knows is coming.

Claire helped me into the gown. My hands were shaking so bad I couldn't get the damn gloves on. She steadied me. "You'll be fine."

"And if I am not?"

"I'll be here…" When the elevator doors opened on the ninth floor, I could already hear the muffled crying. That sound, that specific kind of grief that seeps through walls, it's unmistakable.

I was the last one there. Calvin was by the bed, his daughters, Cathy and Melissa, sitting in the corner, whispering to each

211

other as if this were some surreal sleepover. "Why are they smiling?" I hissed to Claire.

She looked at me softly. "They're kids, Tad. They don't understand what this means yet." I took a deep breath, braced myself, and walked through the door.

It hit me like a wave, not going to lie. I wasn't ready for this. Emma was standing over Mom, over *KK*, as she always called her, holding a rosary, her voice thick and trembling. "Oh, KK," she wailed. "Oh, my sweet Mama."

And just like that, it became a funeral before she was even gone. Emma led the prayers, *Our Father*, *Hail Mary*, and a dozen more I'd forgotten long ago. I mumbled along, lost somewhere between ritual and disbelief. Everyone was crying, everyone except the hospital staff, who had the glazed eyes of people who've seen this scene a thousand times before.

And Mama. She wasn't crying either.

It was hard to even recognize her beneath all the hospital trappings. Tubes, wires, gloves, her arms so fragile they looked like paper left out in the rain. She'd been intubated, her skin pale and bruised, her chest rising and falling like it took effort to stay tethered here.

"Touch her face, Tad," Emma said, voice breaking.

I hesitated. Looked at the doctor. He nodded. "It's okay. She needs that now."

So I did. I reached out, careful as if she'd shatter under my hand, and pressed my palm against her cheek. "Hey, Mama," I whispered. "It's Tad. I love you. We all love you."

Claire stood quietly beside me, a hand on my shoulder. One by one, everyone followed suit. Calvin, Barbara, Georgia, Greg.

Each taking their turn, each saying the same thing in different ways: *I love you. You can go now.*

The doctors moved around us. One of them, the one who seemed to be in charge, finally turned to us after a hushed conversation with the nurses. "It's time," he said. "Are you ready?"

No one ever is. But I heard myself say, "I guess we have to be." They began removing the oxygen. The hiss of the machine faded, replaced by something much heavier: silence. Then came the descent. Her body fought; was it a reflex or an instinct, whatever you want to call it? Every gasp felt like a battle. Her chest rose, fell, rose again.

Emma led us in "Amazing Grace." We stumbled through the verses, voices cracking. Then the *Hail Marys* started again as if the repetition could hold her here just a little longer. I turned to the nurse. "Is our mom dying?" The words came out flat, almost detached.

She looked at me gently. "Yes, Mr. Jaehrling. Your mother is actively dying."

And that was it. The moment everything tilted. The breaths came slower, spaced apart like a clock running out of seconds. Then they stopped. Then started again. False hope. The cruelest kind.

And then, at 5:56 p.m., Katherine Rankin Jaehrling exhaled for the last time. The room stayed still.

Even the machines seemed to pause. Emma whispered another prayer, clutching the rosary. Calvin held Barbara's hand. The girls went silent.

And Claire stepped closer, slipped her hand into mine. Her eyes were red, but she didn't cry the way the others did. She just looked at me with that steady calm, the kind that says, *I'm right here. You're not alone in this.*

I pressed her hand against my chest, where it hurt the most. "Stay," I whispered.

"I'm not going anywhere," she said. And she didn't.

We stood there until the nurses gently ushered us out. And as I turned back one last time, at my mom's still face, the quiet hum of machines now meaningless, I thought about all the years I'd wasted trying to run from this place, this family, this love that terrified me.

I realized something about myself; it was never Houston I was afraid of. It was saying goodbye.

Chapter Twenty Three

In the days and weeks after someone dies, nobody really knows what the hell to do. People pretend they do, of course, all those casseroles and polite murmurs of *"call me if you need anything."* But the real, God's honest truth? Nobody knows. Do we mourn? Pray? Sort out bills? Sit in the dark and stare at old photographs?

What in God's green earth are we supposed to *do*?

For me, the answer came dressed in logistics. Plan the funeral. Contact the church. Make sure the eulogy's in the paper. Write the damn eulogy. And of course, I'd have to give it.

That part, oddly, didn't scare me. I liked giving speeches. I'd never admit it to anyone, but it's the truth. I have what I call the Sally Field Syndrome. *"You like me, you really, really like me."* Yeah. That one. I gave up acting years ago, but apparently, the need for applause never quite left the bloodstream. So, giving the eulogy for my mom, Kitty Jaehrling, didn't seem like a bad gig. But apparently, not everyone saw it that way.

I heard through the family grapevine (Calvin, of course) that I was "making it about myself again." Well, maybe I was. Maybe I wasn't. But what else was I supposed to do with all that grief, turn it into a mime act?

Claire came with me down to Houston. Said she wanted to be there, "for moral support." I pretended I didn't need it, but her presence kept me sane. She was steady, that kind of quiet that doesn't demand anything. We took the four-hour drive in silence for long stretches. She watched the horizon while I replayed old memories like bad reruns: Mom scolding me for tracking mud in, Mom crying after Dad died, Mom smiling in the kitchen like she'd just remembered something funny.

When we got out of the car, Emma greeted me with her usual burst of affection. "Hey, Taddy Boy, great to see you." She hugged me, hard. There was something sad and scared behind her eyes, though. You could feel that same energy in the house as well. It clung to the walls like humidity. Even the sign in the kitchen, "Bless this house and all who enter," felt tired.

I caught Claire reading it and smirking softly. "Bless his house," she said, under her breath, "You might need that one."

"Yeah," I replied, "put me on the prayer list."

We met with Janet Creigh, the woman orchestrating the funeral, and Pastor Richard, who laid out the plan: order of service, who says what, when, and how long. I nodded, pretending to listen, while my brain drifted somewhere else.

There was an election coming up, and the world felt like a pressure cooker. I don't know what possessed me, maybe grief, maybe caffeine, but I started in, "Anyone who votes for that idiot is out of their damn mind."

The look on Roxy's face could've frozen hell over. "Tad," she hissed, "remember to be nice."

"I *am* nice." Her raised eyebrow said otherwise. Claire just shook her head. Later, a man carrying flowers wandered in asking for the Baker Room. I volunteered to lead him, anything to move, to do something.

When I came back, I started ranting again about politics. Couldn't help myself. The room went tense. Claire, sitting across from me, caught my eye and gave this subtle shake of her head, not angry, not judging, just *enough* to pull me back. I shut up. For about five minutes.

216

Then Pastor Richard arrived, saving everyone from me. "Alright," he said, clapping his hands, "it's time."

We filed into the sanctuary. It looked just as I remembered, burgundy carpet splitting the pews, the big bronze cross gleaming up front, the choir seats empty but waiting. It was exactly how Mom would've wanted it. Guests trickled in. I recognized a few faces. Not as many as I'd hoped, though. Some people just can't handle death, or maybe they just couldn't handle *me*. Then the service started.

Pastor Richard spoke first. Then it was my turn. Roxy patted my leg like I was about to perform a monologue at a middle-school talent show. I stood, adjusted my tie, and started.

I talked about Mom's kindness, her stubbornness, her laugh that could fill a room. I wove in the memories my family members had sent me, little things like her humming while she cooked, or how she'd always leave an extra light on "just in case."

I even managed to make them laugh near the end. "We prayed over her, saying the Lord's Prayer and the Hail Mary," I said, pausing just long enough for timing. "Wait, is that right? I think 'Hail Mary' is a football term. I'm not Catholic!"

Laughter. A bit awkward, sure, but laughter nonetheless. I'll take it.

When it was over, I closed with, "Our mom, Kitty, above all, would've wanted us to live fully. So, I hope to see everyone at the reception- Eat something, drink something, and tell stories. She'd have loved that."

I sat down. Roxy patted my knee again. "Good job." Claire leaned in, whispering, "She'd be proud." For a second, I believed her.

217

Following the service, I felt like I was on a roll. The eulogy had landed, people laughed, some even cried. That's a good ratio, right? I could almost feel Mom smirking somewhere, half-proud, half-annoyed that I'd made it a performance. By the time we moved to the reception hall, I was buzzing. Cookies, sandwiches, coffee, I went for all of it. Especially the coffee. Maybe it was the caffeine, but I felt alive again. And then, because I'm apparently incapable of letting a decent mood breathe for five whole minutes, I decided to talk about politics again.

No idea why. Grief? Habit? Maybe I just needed to feel right about something.

"That candidate's a damn moron," I said, mid-sip. "And whoever votes for them is one too."

A woman nearby, I think one of Calvin's in-laws, shot me a polite church smile. "It's not quite that simple, dear."

"With all due respect," I said, topping off my coffee, "we'll have to agree to disagree."

Roxy swooped in like a hawk. "Tad? I think you need another sandwich," she said, already piling one on a plate for me. Then she leaned close and whispered, "Time and place, hon. Time and place."

Claire was across the room, talking to Emma, but I caught her looking over. She didn't say a word. Just raised an eyebrow like a gentle stop sign. I didn't stop. There were plenty of people at the reception, Calvin and his family, some of his friends, a couple of his ex-wives' mothers-in-law (don't even ask). And me, the loudest one in the room, holding court with a cup of Folgers and an inflated sense of moral authority.

Then I started on Al.

"Big oil man, huh?" I said to no one in particular. "If he's such a big oil man, where's the money? Where is it, huh?"

Calvin rolled his eyes so hard I thought they might detach. I think he said something, or maybe he didn't; either way, the message was clear. I was being inappropriate. Again. People began to drift out, polite excuses and empty cups in hand. I grabbed one more coffee for the road, liquid dignity, and headed out into the furnace that is August in Houston.

Good God. The heat hit me right on the front. I'd forgotten how the air down here sticks to you, crawls under your clothes like guilt.

Calvin pulled up beside me as I was unlocking my car. "See you back at the house," he said.

"You mean your house?"

"No, your house."

"Oh."

And there it was, the miscommunication, the tiny spark that always ignites into a full-blown family wildfire. Getting into the car was a whole ordeal. With the MS, some days I move like a drunk man in a dark room. I twisted wrong, lost my balance, and slammed into the steering wheel. It locked. "Oh, hell," I muttered. "Not today."

It had happened before. Usually, if I just drove it out, it loosened. So, I did.

By the time I pulled up to my house, I'd built an entire courtroom drama in my head, starring me, wronged party of one, versus the ungrateful rest of the world. Why were they meeting at *my* house? Who decided that? Who the hell gave Calvin authority to set the agenda in *my* space?

By the time I walked inside, I was fuming.

"WHO ARE YOU," I yelled, "to decide when we meet up at *MY* house?!"

Calvin looked up, startled. "Come on, Tad. Georgia wanted to get Mom's mirror."

"I'm the executor!" I shot back. "I'll decide who gets what and when!"

I snatched the mirror from Georgia's hands. She bolted, literally ran, out to her car. The room gasped like someone had dropped a gun. Calvin called his wife, I called Roxy, and Emma just shook her head.

Roxy picked up. "Hon, calm down. It's not that big of a deal."

"It's a huge deal."

"It's *not,* Tad. Hand the phone to your brother." I did. I have no idea what she said to him, but whatever it was, Calvin deflated a little. He handed the phone back.

"Tad," she said gently, "hun, you gotta calm down, okay?"

"Okay," I said, though I didn't mean it.

"I'll take care of this. Call you when I leave. Love you."

"Love you, too." When I hung up, the silence was awful.

Calvin finally spoke. "What's the deal, Tad? You always do this."

"Do what?"

"Freak out." He was crying now. My brother, who rarely showed anything. "The kids just wanted a few things from Mom. That's all. Why are you being such an asshole?"

And, I swear to God, something in me just snapped. "You're right," I said, voice cracking. "You're totally right. I'm an asshole. A total dick. You wanna hit me? Go ahead, take a swing."

"What?"

"I said hit me! I deserve it."

"Jesus, Tad, you're crazy." Greg, his son, stepped in. "That's my dad you're talking to."

"Greg, I get it. I've been a dick. Go ahead, hit me too."

"Tad, dude," he said quietly, "chill out."

Then Emma lost it. "ENOUGH! Both of you!" she shouted. "Your mother just died, and this is how you're behaving? Calm down. NOW."

"But…"

"LEAVE IT!" And that was that. Emma had this power; she could part family chaos like Moses parting the Red Sea.

We sat down.

Calvin stared at me for a long minute, then spoke softly. "You scared them off, Tad. Georgia's in her car because she's afraid of what you might do. Greg's upset too."

I didn't have an answer.

Claire appeared in the doorway. I didn't even know she'd followed me back from the reception. She looked around the wreckage of my family and said nothing for a long moment. Then she came over, set a hand on my shoulder.

"Tad," she said quietly, "grief makes people do strange things. You're not the only one hurting." I wanted to argue. I wanted to defend myself, to justify it all.

"I am going for a walk… I am giving you time to do what feels right. Okay. Meet you in a while."

Just great. I sighed and went to Greg. I looked at him and asked, "Was I really that bad?" He nodded. "You gotta stop doing this, man."

I laughed. "Well, I can make it up." I walked over to the front door and swung it open. "Georgia, come on in. I want you to have that mirror." She hesitated, but I shoved it into her hands anyway. Then I turned to Greg. "And you, take whatever you'd like."

"Tad, you've *got* to stop doing this if you want to keep hanging out with us," Calvin said, voice clipped. "You keep saying you'll change, and you never do." He sighed. "Look, we gotta go. Come on, Greg." We did the awkward hug thing, those fake 'I love yous' that sound like goodbyes dressed as promises, and then they were gone.

Emma lingered, watching me like someone trying to figure out if the person in front of them was salvageable or already lost. "Look, Tad," she said softly. "I know everyone's hurting, but you can't do this. Your dad's gone, and your mom's gone. All your brother and you have is each other. You can't keep fighting like this."

I looked at her, words stuck in my throat. If she only knew what it felt like inside this chest that's been cracked open for years and never properly sewn shut. If she could just *see* the miserable storm behind my eyes, she'd know why I act this way. I'm crying inside, for the love I never had. And it hurts so fucking bad.

Hurting people hurt others. And suddenly, it all made sense. All of it.

Emma touched my shoulder. "Look, I gotta go. My mom needs help with some things. You gonna be okay?"

"Yes, Emma," I said. "I promise I will. I'll behave."

"You better," she warned. "Or I'm gonna smack you."

And she would, too. I could tell.

After she left, the house felt cavernous. Oh, calm the sadness in my heart. God, I felt so sad. That kind of sadness that doesn't just sit; it spreads. The kind where you want to curl up in a corner and cry until your bones ache, and you want someone, anyone, to come find you and tell you it's gonna be okay. But deep down, you know it won't. So you just cry. And hope for something. Which, honestly, I hadn't done in a long damn time.

I went to the back bedroom and started peeling off my clothes: jacket, trousers, shirt, laying them neatly over the chair. I was heading for the bathroom when I heard it, "Hello? Hello? Tad?"

Roxy's voice. I froze.

"Nice house," she said, like it was an afterthought. "Let's go to the beach!"

"What?"

"Come on, let's go to the beach. You *need* this!"

"Tonight? It's gonna be late by the time we get there."

"It's okay, Tad. I got you. I'm driving. Michelle's coming too."

"Michelle?"

"You know, Michelle, from Rachel's party. Now come on. Snap-snap! Get dressed. We're going." There's something about Roxy's energy; it's chaos wrapped in charm. You can't say no to her.

So I didn't. I threw on a t-shirt, shorts, and my old tennis shoes.

When Michelle showed up, there were hugs and air kisses, and then we were off.

"Who-hoo! Come on, Tad, we're gonna have a great time!" Roxy shouted as we hit the freeway.

Michelle laughed. She had this sharp, sassy energy that could slice through anything fake. She reminded me of Roxy and of who I wished I'd been when I was younger. We talked about everything: love lives, broken promises, what made our hearts sing, the kind of deep stuff people say when they're half high on nostalgia and night air. I brought up politics once, and Roxy shot me a look. "You gotta stop bringing that up, Tad. Not everyone agrees with you, and that's okay. Learn to respect other opinions." She wasn't wrong.

They played country music on the radio. I used to hate it, but something about the twang had started to grow on me. Maybe it was the honesty. The drive stretched out and unfolded into something comforting. Downtown, then past the Beltway, through South Houston, and finally across the causeway. The salt hit the air before I saw the water.

Galveston.

We passed those old mansions, the ones that still looked proud even after being battered by storms for a century. Roxy gave me the rundown, how the great hurricane of 1900 killed six thousand people and crushed the city's future, how Houston rose from its ashes. She told it like a parable. Maybe that's what it was.

"There's this great place down here," she said, grinning. "They sell crabs, burgers, fish, whatever you want." We went.

The restaurant overlooked the water. The moon hung low and fat over the waves, throwing its reflection; it looked as if silver confetti was scattered across the gulf. Ships blinked in the distance.

"It's peaceful out here," Roxy said.

"It is," Michelle added.

Then a bird dropped one right on the railing near us.

"Well," Roxy laughed, "it's the beach."

We ordered. Joked with the waiter. I was supposed to be on a diet, but screw it. I'd already ruined that with the beer earlier, so what was the point? I looked out at the water and sighed. "I really fucked up today, didn't I?"

Roxy shook her head. "You've had a lot going on, hun. That's why I wanted to bring you here. Just relax, okay?"

"Okay." We talked, laughed, let the night stretch around us. Then came that quiet lull that always signals the end.

"Let's go chase some crabs," Roxy said suddenly.

"Crabs?"

"Yes, baby, crabs! I brought the kids here last weekend, and they loved it."

So off we went, Roxy, Michelle, and me, back to the car, then across the highway to the sand. The air was thick with salt and wind and something almost holy.

"Let's take off our shoes!" Roxy shouted.

"What if we step on a crab?" I asked.

"We won't," Michelle said.

I shrugged. "Oh, well. What the heck."

And that was it, barefoot under the moon, chasing shadows on the sand. The night was everything I didn't know I needed.

Roxy shouting, "Oops! I almost got one!" Michelle cackling in the background. Me, some 50-something man running barefoot across the wet sand, pretending the world hadn't broken my heart in twenty different ways.

It was stupid, childish, perfect.

"I brought some blankets," Roxy said. "Y'all wanna lie down?"

We did. We lay flat on our backs, looking up at the stars like they were new. The air was warm, the waves hummed low and lazy. "I love the beach," Roxy said softly.

I turned my head toward the horizon, wondering if forgiveness floated somewhere out there, if my brother might ever see me without all the noise. "You think Calvin'll ever forgive me?" I asked quietly.

"He will, honey," Roxy said. "You just gotta give it time." I wanted to believe her. I really did.

We chased a few more crabs, laughed with some strangers, then packed it up. That long drive back from Galveston always hit me hard, the kind where you start out feeling infinite and end up staring out the window, wondering where your life went sideways. By the time Roxy dropped me off, dawn was crawling over the roofs.

When I stepped inside, the house was still. Then I saw her. Claire was sitting on the couch, one leg folded under her, a book open in her hands. She looked up, startled, like she hadn't expected me back yet.

"Hey," she said softly.

"Hey," I replied, kicking off my shoes. My feet were coated in sand. She closed her book, marking her page with a little pressed flower; trust Claire to have something like that lying around. "You look... better."

"Do I?"

"A little humidly muddy. But better."

I chuckled. "Roxy dragged me to the beach. Said it'd fix me."

"And did it?"

"Maybe halfway." I sat down on the edge of the armchair, elbows on knees. "Rest of the fixing might take a miracle."

She tilted her head, studying me with that calm patience that made me want to both stay and bolt. "You smell like salt water and fried shrimp."

"Yeah," I said. "Guess I needed both."

Claire smiled, but her eyes stayed steady on me. "You're not running forever, Tad. You know that, right?"

"Feels like I've been running my whole damn life."

She set the book aside and patted the space beside her. "Then maybe it's time to sit for a minute." So I did. We didn't talk much after that. Just sat there, her flipping through pages again, me staring at the morning light sneaking through the blinds. It was one of those quiet moments that doesn't fix anything, but makes the ache a little more bearable.

Later, when I finally crashed in bed, I slept hard. Dreamt of waves, of laughter, of my mom's voice somewhere I couldn't quite reach. When I woke, the sunlight was sharp, and there was a knock at the door.

"Tad? Are you naked?" Emma's voice cut through the fog.

"What?"

"Too late," she said, stepping right in and plopping down in the chair.

"You know, Tad, you've got to get this thing right with your brother."

I sighed, rubbing my eyes. "Yeah, I know."

"Your mama won't be at peace till you do."

"I get it," I said. "Claire told me the same thing last night, right before I left."

Emma nodded, satisfied. "Then maybe you should listen to her." She left, and the house went quiet again. I laid in bed for a bit longer than I intended to, still half in a dream, before getting up and grabbing my keys.

The drive back to Dallas was long, but Claire made it bearable. I stopped more than once. Not for gas or food, just to sit on the hood, breathe, and remember everything that had occurred during Kitty's final departure.

Her absence led to an awareness. It made me open a door within myself, and I could see myself in a slightly different light. I know I had to fix a lot of things in me. I had to take accountability for my words and actions.

I had to rectify a lot of things even though I didn't want to.

Chapter Twenty Four

The days after Mama's funeral were a blur of paperwork and emotions. I didn't feel like having lawyers, signatures, banks, or family. Everyone had an opinion; everyone thought they were the executor of her soul. There were assets to divide, accounts to close, assets to inventory, and people to appease. All that sentimental crap about "healing" it gets really thin when you're staring at financial statements and probate forms.

The only thing that made me feel even remotely useful was knowing that at least I'd helped keep Mama's affairs from turning into a disaster. When I first got involved, she was down to less than six hundred thousand liquid, plus the house. Her assets were stuck with some bank's trust department charging 1.5% a year to underperform the market; all in mutual funds with a bad allocation, no growth. Typical.

"She should be all stock," I'd told my dad. Al agreed, mostly because I was louder about it. We moved her account to the brokerage where I was working, sold the mutuals, bought decent positions, and cut distributions for a bit. It worked.

Then Al had one of his "brainstorms," which usually meant he'd just had a cup of strong coffee.

"Let's put the house in a trust," he said. "That way, no smooth-talker from the senior center convinces her to sell it." I'll give him that one. It was smart. But the distributions, over a hundred grand a year from a six-hundred-thousand-dollar portfolio and a four-hundred-thousand-dollar house; that was insane.

229

"Mmm-mmm-mmm," I muttered one day, staring at the spreadsheet. "This is never gonna work." Al, of course, disagreed. The fights were legendary.

"How do you EXPECT Calvin and me to pay for this when Mama runs out of money, huh?"

"Tad, calm down," he'd say, which of course made me not calm down. "Let me think about it."

He'd think. I'd stew. But I was prepared. I'd learned that sometimes the best way to win a battle is to make someone else believe they came up with your plan themselves. So I went to one of our brokers and this was all before the Al calling me incident. This is how it played out.

"You want me to what?" the guy asked.

"Create a report," I said, "that shows everything, the trust, the house, current annual expenses and send it to my dad."

Three weeks later, my phone rang.

"Tad, can Kitty move into your house? Emma can move in, of course."

"My gosh, Dad, wow! Are you serious? That's a brilliant idea!"

He puffed up through the phone. "Thanks, son. I think it's the best way to handle this."

"I agree, Dad. I'm so pleased that *you* thought of this."

Boom. Game, set, and match to Tad. The art of manipulation is not getting your way. It's getting someone to think your way *was theirs*. I could've taught a class.

After all that, the paperwork, the trust setup, the distributions finally aligned, the money would last.

But then came the internment ceremony. Mama's ashes in the columbarium. Another drive to Houston. Another round of family tension and unspoken resentments.

Barbara, my sister-in-law, (who was often quite annoyed with me) would be there, which meant the air would be thick enough to slice. I made the four-hour drive, quick stop at Bucee's because some habits you don't break, then stayed overnight at my old house in Houston. Still couldn't bring myself to sleep in the middle bedroom, the room Mom had been using.

The service was supposed to be at 1:30. At least that's what I remembered. But first, the walk. I *had* to get my sanity in somehow, and Memorial Park had been my ritual for years, my moving meditation, my way to talk myself down from whatever mountain I'd built that week. So I threw on shorts and a t-shirt and went.

I don't run anymore. Not since the balance issues got worse. MS has a way of humbling you like that, strips you of speed and grace till you're just a guy doing a brisk walk, pretending it's a choice. Still, I wasn't one of those 60-year-old ladies you see at the mall flailing their arms like windmills. No. I walked like a normal person. Because, dammit, I *am* a normal person. At least, that's what I told myself.

Halfway through the loop, my watch buzzed. I glanced down. Hell. I was running late. I picked up the pace. A little jog, then faster, the Houston humidity pressing in on me like a wet towel. I could see my car up ahead, parked by a ditch.

Now, I could've taken the long way around, added another minute, maybe two, but no. Impatient idiot that I am, I decided to cut through the ditch.

Bad move. My foot slipped, and down I went. Face first. Instinct kicked in, and I threw out my left foot to catch myself. Saved my face, sacrificed my toe.

"Fuck," I hissed, rolling onto my back. My left big toe was screaming. God, I hate multiple sclerosis. The way it steals coordination, balance, pride, one stupid movement at a time. But I got up, limped to the car, and drove home. No time for a shower. Emma had already left to pick up her friend. I'd meet them there. I yanked on the same suit I'd worn to the funeral, shirt half-wrinkled, no tie. Too hot for one anyway.

1:15. My phone rang. Calvin.

"Tad, are you on the way?"

"I'm almost there. I'm on time, though."

"No, Tad. It started at one. Remember?" I didn't. Because I never actually *read* the texts. I skim. I nod. I move on. I opened the thread. And there it was, plain as day. *1:00 p.m.*

"Good one, Tad," I muttered. "Real attentive."

I sped the rest of the way, heart pounding, toe throbbing.

Calvin called again to guide me in. I parked, stepped out, trying to ignore the pain in my foot. Everyone was already waiting, eyes on me as if I were the kid who showed up late to his own graduation.

And there it was again, that mix of love, tension, and exhaustion that seems to define every Rankin-Jaehrling gathering. I plastered on my best 'everything's fine' smile, limped toward them, and muttered under my breath:

"Always the goddamn ditch."

The air that afternoon was so thick you could chew it. Not just with heat, but with silence. If you'd had an ice pick handy, you could've chipped at the tension, but it would've taken more than that to make a dent.

Barbara wouldn't look at me. Emma sighed that polite little sigh of hers and tried for a smile that didn't quite land. Her friend Bonnie waved cheerfully like we were at a Sunday barbecue instead of an internment. Calvin and Greg were too overly cordial as if hinting, *We're pretending everything's fine until you leave.*

The rest of the family just stood there, silent, staring at the little black urn like it might explode.

Pastor Richard, who'd preached so beautifully at Mom's funeral, started speaking, doing his best "gentle shepherd" routine. A few words about faith, peace, ashes to ashes. He meant well, but it all sounded like white noise against the beating sun. Then came the part I always dread, *"Does anyone else have a few words they'd like to share?"*

Of course, Bonnie stepped up. She always does. She said something sweet and harmless, bless her heart, the kind of thing you forget thirty seconds later but feel obligated to nod at. Then silence again. I looked around, waiting for someone else to say something. Emma, maybe, or one of the kids. Hell, even Calvin. But nothing. Just the sound of a hot wind rattling the tent above us.

So, me being me, I opened my big mouth.

"You know," I said, stepping forward a little, "as the oldest, I lived with her for seven years before my brother was born. Dad was at work most of the time, so I got to see firsthand what a great woman my mom was." The second the words left my

233

mouth, I could feel the temperature drop ten degrees. You could've heard a pin drop on that manicured grass.

Barbara froze. Emma looked at her shoes. Pastor Richard smiled that awkward, church-approved smile that says *I'm not touching this with a ten-foot pole.*

"Thank you, Tad," he said, voice cracking just slightly. "Does... anyone else have anything to add?"

Nope. Just the wind and the rustle of polyester suits.

He cleared his throat. "Alright then. Calvin, Tad... if you'll help me, we can place the ashes." Calvin hesitated for half a beat. I didn't. If nothing else, I'd be first this time. I took the urn from the pastor's hands, and Calvin followed me to the columbarium. The marble wall was cool, impersonal, exactly how it should be. We slid the urn in, side by side, our mom's entire life now condensed to a few pounds of dust.

Silence again. No one said a damn word. Barbara stood off to the side, staring straight ahead like she could see through the wall, through all of us.

Finally, Pastor Richard sighed, probably deciding we were a lost cause. "Uh... well," he said, "I'll let you all spend some time here. Tad, Calvin, I'll need to talk with you both later to handle some paperwork." And with that, he left us standing there; a family in name, strangers in practice.

After a minute, I broke the spell. "Well," I said, my voice too loud, "I guess it's time to go."

Chapter Twenty Five

People started drifting off. The chatter was low, uneasy, as if everyone was relieved it was over but too polite to show it. The columbarium gleamed in the sun, those tidy white walls holding so many stories sealed behind brass plates. Ours just got one more.

Calvin and Greg murmured about something I couldn't catch. Emma was holding her friend Bonnie's hand, nodding absently. The nieces hugged me, little arms clinging as if I might disappear if they let go. Kids always forgive faster than adults. They don't carry the history, the grudges, the what-ifs. They just feel what's right in front of them.

Barbara didn't hug me. When I turned to her, she pivoted just slightly, but enough. Her gaze fixed straight ahead on the grass. Not even a flicker. Her silence could've frozen fire. So, naturally, I tried to fill the void. "So... what's everybody doing for lunch?" My voice sounded too bright, too forced. I heard it, even if no one else said a word.

Calvin cleared his throat. "Barbara, Tad says he wants to go to lunch."

"I'm not hungry," she said, crisp as a knife. She didn't even look my way. She got into her black Suburban, slammed the door hard enough for the sound to echo off the marble. Then she rolled down the window a few inches, just enough to send a message.

"Calvin, can you come here for a minute? I need to talk to you."

Calvin went, slow and steady. They talked in low tones, her gestures sharp, every flick of her hand aimed my way. I didn't need to hear the words. I'd been in that courtroom before. When he came back, he had that calm, deliberate look he always used when he was about to say something that mattered.

"Hey, brother," he said. "I need to talk with you for a sec."

"Sure," I said, bracing like I was about to take a punch.

He rubbed his hands together, glanced at the ground, then right into me. "You know, the kids idolize you. They're always talking about Uncle Tad this, Uncle Tad that." His voice softened, but it didn't waver. "But these angry outbursts, they've gotta stop."

I blinked, trying to buy time. "What are you talking about?"

He tilted his head. "Come on, Tad. I thought you were supposed to be getting better. You keep saying you won't do it again, but then you do. I try to keep you included, to make you part of things, but if this keeps up…" He exhaled through his nose. "I don't know, man. I can't keep defending you." The words landed hard. I felt every one.

I swallowed, hard. "I'm sorry," I said, voice barely more than a rasp. "I don't know what happened. Something just… got into me, and I couldn't stop."

He nodded slowly, lips pressed tight. "You've gotta stop, man. You're my brother, and I love you. But you've gotta stop. We shouldn't be at war with each other."

That last line cracked something open. We hugged, not one of those back-slapping, perfunctory ones either. It was an awkward long hug. The kind of hug that says, *I still love you, but damn, you make it hard.* When he stepped back, I realized everyone else was gone. Just us and the wind kicking up the

236

dry grass around the graves. I watched him walk toward Barbara's car. She didn't even glance back.

That's when I saw her. Claire.

She was sitting on one of the stone benches near the walkway, a slim paperback open in her lap, like she'd been there a while. I didn't even notice her before was too caught up in my own head. She must've come back after her walk. She didn't say anything right away, just looked up, the corners of her eyes soft with something that wasn't pity. Something closer to knowing.

"You okay?" she asked.

"Define okay." I tried to joke, but my voice cracked halfway through.

She set the book down beside her and stood. The wind tugged at her dress, that faint floral pattern shifting like ripples on water. When she came closer, she reached out and took my hand.

Her fingers were cool. "I heard what Calvin said," she murmured.

I looked down. "Yeah. He wasn't wrong."

"No," she said quietly. "He wasn't."

We stood there like that for a while, the silence stretching. I kept staring at the spot where Barbara's Suburban had been. It felt like every word I'd said in the past week was still hanging in the air between us.

Claire squeezed my hand, just enough to make me look at her. "Then choose us," she whispered.

"Us?"

She nodded. "Me. This. Whatever good you've still got left in you. Stop feeding the fire, Tad. Let it die out. You don't need it anymore." Her voice was calm, but there was an edge of plea in it, not desperation, just care that had seen too much. I couldn't answer. Not right away. I just looked at her. The faint lines at the edges of her eyes. The way she bit her lip when she was scared to say too much. She didn't let go.

Finally, I nodded. "Okay," I said. "I'll try." She gave me that half-smile she always did when she didn't quite believe me but wanted to.

We walked back toward the truck, our shadows long and thin on the pavement. The sun was lower now, bleeding orange across the lot. I opened her door first. She slid in, quiet, hands folded in her lap. The drive home was silent, except for the hum of tires on the road. Every so often, she'd glance my way, but she didn't press. She knew pushing me would just make me shut down.

When we got to the house, she went inside while I stayed in the driveway. The sky was going dim, all bruised purple and silver clouds. I just sat there, engine running, hands still gripping the wheel.

My phone buzzed. A message from Calvin.

"You'll always be my brother." I stared at it, reread it, then let the phone drop into my lap.

Always my brother. Yeah. Maybe. If I didn't burn that bridge next.

I turned off the ignition, leaned my head back against the seat, and finally exhaled. The house lights were on. Through the front window, I could see Claire moving around, probably setting the kettle on, maybe lighting one of those candles she

238

likes that smells like vanilla and cedar. Domestic peace. Stability. Things I never thought I'd want until I almost lost them.

Maybe she was right. Maybe it was time to choose *us*.

But the thing about fires, they don't just die because you tell them to. You've gotta stand there and watch the smoke, and live with the smell it leaves behind.

Chapter Twenty Six

God, I loved this place. Nature at its best, beautiful scenery, and on most days, I see beautiful people too. I'd been here so many times that it's somewhat a place of comfort, or maybe something better than home. But I didn't feel that today.

A recent renovation had changed things; I noticed widened trails, added signs, and rerouted a few loops that didn't need rerouting. They called it an "extension," said it was now *officially* three miles instead of "supposedly" three. I wasn't sure who measured it before, but someone had apparently lied by half a mile.

The city or maybe the parks department had sent out one of those polite little letters asking if folks like me wanted to "contribute to the project." Meaning: pay for it. Ever the penny-pincher, I'd politely declined and parked on the street. Some habits die hard.

It was a good day for November. Cool but not cold, sky the color of faded denim. Houston wasn't known for winter. Every year, the cold fronts tried to make their way in, some from the Pacific, some from up north, and every once in a while, one of those full-blown Canadian blasts that made everyone lose their minds and buy bread. Then, of course, there were the polar vortexes; the rare, vicious ones.

I kind of liked those, if I'm honest. They helped me pretend I was somewhere else. Somewhere that had seasons, maybe a place where people drank cocoa and wore sweaters without irony. They made me forget I was in Houston, where it could easily be seventy degrees on Christmas morning and everyone still pretended it was festive.

But November wasn't for that kind of cold. November was for gray skies and soft light, for that little in-between space before the year gave out. Today was just that, forty-something degrees, no rain, just the smell of damp earth from the drizzle earlier. Rain was as much a part of southeast Texas as bad traffic and barbecue. The leaves here didn't turn amber or gold or any of those cinematic things. They stayed green until a cold snap turned them brown overnight.

This day felt like so many before it, but it wasn't. Not because of the weather. The weather was doing what it always did. But something in the air was different. Something in *me* was different. I knew that things were changing. Maybe for good. And I hated that. I've always hated change, but that didn't stop it.

I walked along the clay trail, the one I'd tread a thousand times, and it hit me: this could be one of the last times I'd ever walk it like this. Alone, free, unhurried.

"Nice shirt!" someone called, a half-dressed blond guy jogging past, earbuds in, skin glowing with sweat.

Right. The shirt.

The one that said "ENUF." I got comments on it a lot. Most folks thought it meant "enough," as in, *I've had enough.* But it wasn't that. ENUF stood for *Everyone Needs Understanding Friends.*

I hadn't known that until rehab in Dallas. I'd worn it for months, thinking it was just a clever bit of slang. Funny how meanings sneak up on you. Today, though, it felt fitting. Everyone does need understanding friends. Not everyone has them.

I thought about this park again, Memorial Park. The name always struck me as ironic. A park for remembering, sure, but also for escaping memory. I'd done both here. I'd mourned loves lost, both real and imaginary, the kind of grief that made your chest ache for months. I'd walked these trails with that tight, hollow feeling in my ribs, thinking the sadness would never leave. It always does, eventually. But it leaves a dent.

I'd come here searching for connection, belonging, that mythical thing called peace. And, more than anything, love. That's what I wanted most in the world; not money, not status, not even the admiration of strangers. Just someone to hold me and say, *"You're going to be alright, Tad. I love you. Forever."*

That's it. That's all. So why the hell was that the hardest thing to find? I'd loved plenty. Some had loved me back. Some hadn't. I guess that's how life works, but it doesn't make it any easier to accept. Every time I came here, though, I hoped. Even after everything. I thought maybe this park might hand me a second chance.

I used to post about this place all the time on Facebook, back before COVID turned everyone into political philosophers and the world started burning from the inside out.

I'd walked these trails with Joanna once. God, she loved this place. I remember seeing it through her eyes that winter, how green and alive it was, even in the dead months. That relationship ended, like most things do, but the park stayed the same.

The song "Everlasting Love" floated into my head. It always did here. Some old version from a radio hold line years ago. I'd been put on hold and heard it, and for some reason, it stuck. That melody, that idea that something is *everlasting*. What a cruel joke.

Mom was gone. Dad was gone. The job, gone. Emma was packing to move. What now? Was this it?

Was this endless, quiet ache what the rest of my life would feel like? I loved this park, but it also reminded me of everything I didn't have: companionship, clarity, a sense of direction.

The phrase came back to me, like it always did: *a longing sense of melancholy.* I'd thought of it once, walking around some man-made lake in Plano years ago, and it never left me. That's what I felt. Still. A thirst for something I couldn't name and couldn't quench.

Each day blended into the next, the weeks marked only by weekends and the occasional holiday. Life was turning into white noise. And here I was, fifty-six and still middle-aged, because hell- what else was I supposed to call it? But even I could feel it. The slowing down. The creaks in the bones, the early nights, the weight of too much reflection.

I thought back to my thirties, those wild years before *the diagnosis.* Before everything shifted. Back when the parties blurred together and the spotlight still loved me. When I thought success and charm would keep me young forever.

The delusion of perpetuity.

That's what it was. Thinking things would never end. That love, that youth, that energy; it would just keep on going. But things change. You fight it, you cling to what's slipping, but eventually you realize the fight's useless. You just… give in.

The shadows grew longer across the path. The sun was slipping behind the trees, turning everything copper and gold. The park lights blinked on, one by one. I checked my watch. Damn, I was getting late.

Time for dinner. I pulled out my phone and smiled at the name on the screen. Claire. Maybe I'd take her out tonight, and also Emma. She will be leaving soon, and I am going to miss her. Maybe that's what I needed- just some light, some laughter, some reminder that I was still alive.

The moon was rising as I walked back toward the car, the air carrying that sweet, earthy smell of damp leaves and hope.

Yeah. God, I loved this place. Even when it broke my heart.

Chapter Twenty Seven

Emma was in a good mood that night, which surprised me. For someone who'd just lost her best friend, her job, and, soon, her place to live, she carried herself like sunlight in human form. Maybe that was just Emma. No matter how heavy the clouds, she found a way to shine through the cracks. When I walked through the back door, she turned and grinned.

"Tad, look at you. You're too skinny. You're *flacco*."

I laughed. "It's the diet, Emma. Keeps me humble."

She wagged a finger at me. "Some good Mexican food will take care of that."

And just like that, it was decided, Spanish Flowers it would be. The Heights was buzzing that night, full of warm November air and string lights blinking over patios. Spanish Flowers had been there longer than I'd been alive, one of those rare places that had watched the city evolve and refused to apologize for staying the same.

Claire came along too, of course. We were seated quickly, the way regulars often are. Chips, salsa, and familiarity landed on the table at once.

The conversation started with small talk; weather, groceries, the new mural on Yale Street but eventually rolled into deeper things, the kind you only talk about when the company feels like home.

Emma talked about her oldest daughter, who was finally doing well. The youngest, she said, was "still figuring things out." Her grandson had been accepted into a program for autistic adults, she said it with pride, the kind that makes your chest feel warm.

Then she looked at me, her tone softening. "And how are *you*, Tad? What are you gonna do now that your mama's gone? I know she wouldn't want you sitting around here, moping."

I exhaled, half-smile tugging at my lips. "That's the million-dollar question, Emma. I don't really have to work anymore, but I can't just sit around either. So…" I hesitated, but the words felt right. "I think I'm finally gonna finish that book. And you, my friend, are gonna be in it."

Emma's eyes widened. "Me? Really?"

"Yep. Just promise me you'll still talk to me after you read what I write."

She chuckled. "Well, make sure you make me look good."

"Oh, Emma, that's easy. You *are* good. You saved my mom's life, and by extension, you saved me. Don't ever forget that." Her eyes shimmered in the low light. Claire reached across and gave her hand a gentle squeeze. There was something quiet, sacred, about the three of us sitting there like the universe had folded time just enough to let us share that one perfect meal.

The rest of the evening drifted like an old country song filled with nostalgia, a little sadness, but full of love. We talked about the past, the chaos, the good and bad years. We tiptoed around politics, laughed about how different we were, and agreed it didn't matter. Some people let the world tear them apart. We weren't gonna be those people.

After dinner, we drove home under a sleepy Houston sky. The streetlights flickered like memories.

Back at the house, Emma disappeared into her room, still humming. I stood in the hall for a moment, watching her door close, realizing this was probably our last night under the same roof. It hit me harder than I expected. She'd been my anchor, my mom's caretaker, my reminder that goodness still existed in simple acts; laundry folded, tea poured, prayers whispered.

Claire was in the bedroom where we stayed, folding clothes into a duffel.

"I got your notebook," she said, nodding toward the bed. "And snacks for the road."

The trip. Our small writing retreat in New Orleans. A new chapter, literally and otherwise.

I sat beside her, watching her laugh as she tried to zip the overstuffed bag. "You're bringing half the house," I teased.

"You'll thank me when you need socks," she shot back, smiling.

We sat there, side by side, the hum of the old ceiling fan filling the silence. I could feel the weight of everything behind me: loss, change, love, survival, and yet, for once, it didn't crush me. It steadied me.

Writing every day. Living every day. I was still learning, still breaking, still healing, but doing it with someone who saw me as more than my past.

Claire leaned against my shoulder. "You ready for this?"

I nodded. "Yeah. I think I finally am."

Tomorrow, we'd drive east. Emma would move back to her daughter's, and the house would quiet down, maybe too much. But tonight, we were here. Together, existing in that small, golden space between endings and beginnings.

247

I looked around the room and observed- the half-packed bags, Claire's smile, the faint sound of Emma's voice down the hall, and I thought, *This isn't the end.*

No. It wasn't a full stop.

Just a bright, defiant semicolon.

******

Life did turn out for the better. Ten years is the lucky number for me. I am now ten years sober, which is a really big achievement if you ask me. I made it, with the guidance of God and my loved ones, of course. I can't take the whole credit.

And, I would like to give some credit to my resilient spirit, which comes from God. I kept moving forward, stumbled, skinned my knees every now and then, but I kept crawling.

Sometimes, a crawl is enough. Movement is movement, don't you think?

Goodbye and keep moving forward. You will get there. Just keep moving and praying, one Day at a Time until the End comes along. and it always does.

For now.

www.ingramcontent.com/pod-product-compliance
Lightning Source LLC
Chambersburg PA
CBHW071404050426
42335CB00063B/1093